SURGICAL GEMS

In
Dermatology

Edited by
PERRY ROBINS, M.D.

Associate Professor of Clinical Dermatology
New York University School of Medicine
Chief of Mohs Surgery
New York University Medical Center
New York, New York

Journal Publishing Group
New York, New York

Dedicated to Elizabeth and Larry Robins

Director of Publications: Roberta Fineman

Copyeditor: Frances Chapman

Book Design: Howard Roberts

Cover Design: Howard Roberts

Illustrations by: Monika Bittman (pages 4, 7, 9, 11, 12, 16, 17, 27, 29, 33–37, 46, 48, 49, 61, 71, 74, 83, 89, 90, 92, 93, 95, 105, 111, 116)

Howard Roberts (pages 31, 113, 114)

Printed in the United States of America.

Library of Congress Cataloging-in-Publication Data

Surgical gems in dermatology.

   Includes bibliographies and index.
   1. Skin—Surgery—Atlases. 2. Skin—Cancer—Surgery
—Atlases. I. Robins, Perry, 1930–   . [DNLM:
1. Skin—surgery—atlases. 2. Skin Neoplasms—surgery—
atlases. WR 17 S961]
RD520.S87 1988   617'.477   88-31982
ISBN 0-9621300 0-1

CONTRIBUTORS

Jean Arouete, M.D., *Chief, Dermatology Service, Rothschild Foundation, Paris, France.*

Saul Asken, M.D., *Medical Director, Cosmetic Surgery Center of Connecticut, P.C., Westport, Connecticut.*

Samuel Ayres III, M.D., *Associate Clinical Professor of Dermatology, University of Southern California, Los Angeles.*

Robert L. Baran, M.D., *Head, Dermatology Division, General Hospital, Cannes, France.*

Jeffrey H. Binstock, M.D., *Clinical Assistant Professor of Dermatology, University of California Medical School, San Francisco, California.*

Eugene L. Bodian, M.D., F.A.C.P., *Chief, Division of Dermatology, North Shore University Hospital, Long Island; Associate Professor of Dermatology, New York University Medical Center, New York; Clinical Professor of Dermatology, Cornell University Hospital, New York, New York.*

Martin Braun III, M.D., *Associate Clinical Professor, Department of Dermatology, George Washington University, Washington, D.C.*

Janis P. Campbell, M.D., F.R.C.P.(C), *Clinical Lecturer, University of Calgary, Calgary, Alberta, Canada.*

Roger I. Ceilley, M.D., *Assistant Clinical Professor, Department of Dermatology, University of Iowa, Iowa City, Iowa.*

Russell W. Cohen, M.D., *Department of Dermatology, New York University Medical Center, New York, New York.*

Leonard M. Dzubow, M.D., *Assistant Professor, Department of Dermatology, University of Pennsylvania School of Medicine, Philadelphia, Pennsylvania.*

Ervin Epstein, M.D., *Associate Clinical Professor of Dermatology, University of California, San Francisco, California.*

Rafael Falabella, M.D., *Professor, Department of Internal Medicine, Section of Dermatology, Universidad del Valle, Hospital Universitario, Cali, Columbia.*

Lawrence M. Field, M.D., F.I.A.C.S., *Clinical Associate Professor (Dermatologic Surgery), University of California, San Francisco, and Stanford University Medical Center, Stanford, California.*

Richard Gibbs, M.D., *Clinical Professor of Dermatology, New York University Medical Center, New York, New York.*

Richard G. Glogau, M.D., *Associate Clinical Professor, Department of Dermatology, University of California, San Francisco, California.*

Leonard Goldberg, M.D., *Associate Professor of Clinical Dermatology and Chief of Dermatologic Surgery, Baylor College of Medicine, Houston, Texas.*

Eckart Haneke, M.D., *Director, Dermatology Clinic, Wuppertal, West Germany.*

C. William Hanke, M.D., *Professor of Dermatology and Pathology, Indiana University School of Medicine, Indianapolis, Indiana.*

Marwali Harahap, M.D., *Professor, Department of Dermatology, University of North Sumatra School of Medicine, Medan, Indonesia.*

Enrique Hernández-Pérez, M.D., *Professor and Chairman, Section of Dermatology, University of El Salvador School of Medicine, San Salvador, El Salvador.*

Thomas Kohn, M.D., *Lecturer in Dermatology, Jewish General Hospital, McGill University, Montreal, Quebec, Canada.*

Emanuel G. Kuflik, M.D., *Clinical Associate Professor (Dermatology), University of Medicine and Dentistry of New Jersey, New Jersey Medical School, Newark, New Jersey.*

Dan Meirson, M.D., *Department of Dermatology, New York University Medical Center, New York, New York.*

George R. Mikhail, M.D., *Director of Mohs Surgery, Department of Dermatology, Henry Ford Hospital, Detroit, Michigan.*

Ricardo G. Mora, M.D., *is in private practice of Mohs micrographic surgery.*

David S. Orentreich, M.D., *Assistant Clinical Professor, Department of Dermatology, Mount Sinai School of Medicine, New York, New York.*

Norman Orentreich, M.D., *Clinical Professor, Department of Dermatology, New York University School of Medicine, New York, New York.*

James B. Pinski, M.D., F.A.C.P., F.I.C.S., *Associate Clinical Professor of Dermatology, Northwestern University Medical School, Chicago, Illinois.*

Edward F. Pitard, M.D., *Assistant Professor, Department of Dermatology, Louisiana State University School of Medicine, New Orleans, Louisiana.*

John L. Ratz, M.D., F.A.C.P., *Staff Dermatologist, Department of Dermatology, Cleveland Clinic Foundation, Cleveland, Ohio.*

Blas A. Reyes, M.D., *Mohs Surgery Fellow, New York University Medical Center, New York, New York.*

Perry Robins, M.D., *Associate Professor of Clinical Dermatology, New York University School of Medicine, and Chief of Mohs Surgery, New York University Medical Center, New York, New York.*

Annalis Scherrer-Koch, M.D., *is a dermatologic surgeon in private practice in Zurich, Switzerland.*

Samuel J. Stegman, M.D., *Associate Clinical Professor, Department of Dermatology, University of California, San Francisco, California.*

Theodore A. Tromovitch, M.D., *Associate Clinical Professor of Dermatology, University of California, San Francisco, California.*

Walter P. Unger, M.D., F.R.C.P.(C), F.A.C.P., *Assistant Professor of Medicine (Dermatology), University of Toronto, Ontario, Canada.*

Carl Vinciullo, M.B., B.S., F.A.C.D., *Dermatologist, Royal Perth Hospital, Perth, Western Australia.*

Ronald G. Wheeland, M.D., F.A.C.P., *Associate Professor, Department of Dermatology, University of California, Davis Health Sciences Center, Sacramento, California.*

John M. Yarborough, Jr., M.D., *Clinical Professor of Dermatology, Tulane University School of Medicine, New Orleans, Louisiana.*

CONTENTS

PART III—DERMABRASION

PART IV—SURGICAL PROCEDURES OF THE EAR

PART V—SURGICAL PROCEDURES OF THE SCALP

PART VI—NAIL SURGERY

PART VII—SURGICAL AIDS AND INSTRUMENTS

INDEX   117

INTRODUCTION

Over the course of many years of teaching residents, fellows, dermatologists, and other specialists, I am frequently asked, "Isn't there an easier or better way to perform this procedure?" Very often, the answer is "yes!"

It occurred to me that a collection of these practical tips and techniques, which I call "surgical gems," would be useful to all. I also anticipated that many of my colleagues would have surgical gems of their own to contribute. The result of our joint efforts, therefore, is this book, the first in a series.

Some of the techniques described here are original while others are adaptations of procedures that were taught or had been published elsewhere. In all cases, we accepted each gem as an educational contribution. I hope, in the spirit of the free exchange of valuable information with our peers, we will be forgiven any oversights in attribution.

We welcome any suggestions and contributions you wish to make for the next edition of the book. Please send these to *Surgical Gems*, c/o Journal of Dermatologic Surgery and Oncology, 245 Fifth Avenue, New York, NY 10016.

Finally, I want to thank all contributors to this volume and to those now scheduled for Volume II. In particular, my deepest gratitude goes to Drs. Carl Vinciullo, Chaim Kaplan, and Blas Reyes for their invaluable assistance in editing and selecting these gems. Last, and certainly not least, I want to acknowledge the efforts of the late William F. X. Deegan, Publisher of the *Journal of Dermatologic Surgery and Oncology*, for helping to make this book a reality.

—*Perry Robins, M.D.*
Editor

PART I

ANESTHESIA

Anesthesia for Plantar Skin
By Richard Gibbs, M.D.

Anesthetic Injection Technique
By Martin Braun III, M.D., and Leonard M. Dzubow, M.D.

Regional Anesthesia for Facial Collagen Injection
By Thomas Kohn, M.D.

Regional Block Anesthesia of the Ear
By Ronald G. Wheeland, M.D.

ANESTHESIA FOR PLANTAR SKIN
By Richard Gibbs, M.D.

There is a simple trick to painlessly anesthetizing plantar skin when, for example, one prepares to remove a plantar wart. I learned the trick from a podiatrist, Dr. Marvin Steinberg.

TECHNIQUE

The anesthetic should be introduced into the dorsal surface of the foot, the exact site depending upon the location of the area on the sole to be anesthetized (Fig 1).

For example, if a wart is located on the lateral aspect of the sole, one injects the anesthetic into the thin, relatively pain-insensitive dorsolateral skin, raises a bleb, points the needle plantarward, and proceeds to infiltrate the tissue while advancing the needle. Soon the skin on the sole at the site of the infiltration will blanch. Sometimes, the goal has been accomplished, and the plantar lesion has been anesthetized. However, more often, one must further infiltrate the sole to reach a lesion. Since anesthesia has already been obtained on the sole, it is an easy matter to withdraw the syringe and needle, reinsert it into the anesthetized area of the sole, and thread it toward the eventual goal, again injecting while pushing the syringe. Rarely, it may be necessary to withdraw the needle completely and reinsert it a second time to reach the site to be anesthetized.

If a plantar lesion is in the web space or in areas overlying the middle metatarsal heads, it is probably easier to spread the adjacent toes wide apart and inject directly into the web space from the dorsal skin. Advance the needle plantarward until blanching occurs on the sole, and withdraw the needle. Reinsert it, if necessary, into the anesthetized area of the sole, and angle the needle and syringe toward the exact site to be anesthetized, creeping toward it and injecting at the same time (Fig 2).

For the most part, the same principles can be applied to anesthetizing skin on the hand.

The technique takes a few moments more, but it is clearly superior in terms of patient comfort to injecting directly into the volar skin and producing sharp pain.

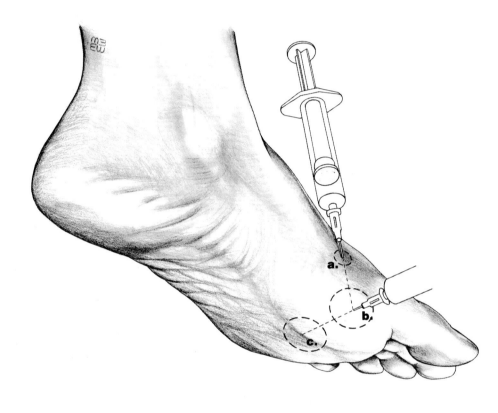

Fig 1. Areas to be anesthetized on the sole (dashed circles). Needle is inserted into the dorsum (A) of the foot and advanced plantarward. The circle at B marks the plantar area anesthetized by injection into dorsal skin. Lesions outside circle at B would require withdrawing the needle and reinserting. To anesthetize the lesion at C would probably require a second withdrawal of the needle.

4 / SURGICAL GEMS: In Dermatology

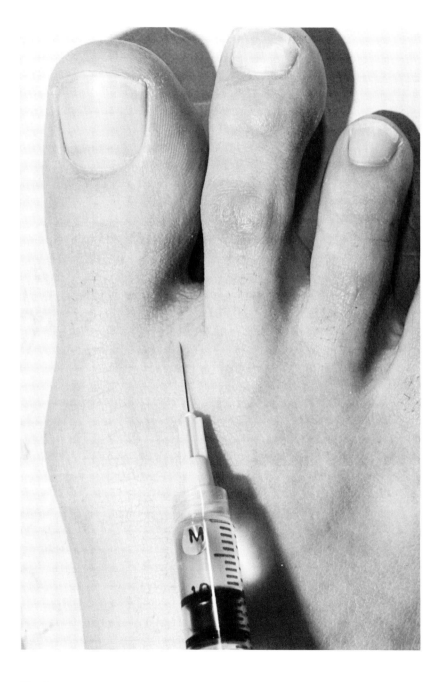

Fig 2.   **Injecting the dorsal aspect of the web space to get to the sole rapidly.**

ANESTHETIC INJECTION TECHNIQUE

By Martin Braun III, M.D., and Leonard M. Dzubow, M.D.

Injection of 1% Xylocaine with epinephrine (Astra) into the nose is often a painful procedure. Once the needle has penetrated the epidermis, pain can be reduced by injecting the anesthetic slowly. However, two techniques can further reduce the discomfort of anesthetic injection.

TECHNIQUES

The pain related to the puncture in the nose can be minimized by inserting the needle directly through one of the more obvious infundibular follicular structures (in this way, there is no puncture through intact skin). Of course, the use of a 30-gauge needle makes a significant contribution to the minimization of pain. When injecting anesthetic into the nose, inject into a plane above the perichondrium into the subcutaneous space below the dermis (Fig 1). Although there may be fewer nerve endings present at this site, a more likely explanation for the lessening of pain is that the volume of fluid in this space creates less pressure and, thus, less stimulation of nerve endings.

In addition, significant discomfort associated with local anesthesia is the sensation of warmth and burning. This sensation is in part due to the acidity of the material, which is necessary to prevent the oxidation of the epinephrine. Fresh Xylocaine and epinephrine can be mixed as needed, so that the solution need not be so acidic. Ten milliliters of 1% Xylocaine can be mixed with 0.1 ml epinephrine solution (1:1,000) to obtain a final concentration of 1% Xylocaine with 1:100,000 epinephrine. The mixture needs to be discarded after 24 hr, since oxidation of the epinephrine is likely to occur after this period. Most patients report that discomfort is reduced by about half with the use of a fresh Xylocaine-and-epinephrine solution.

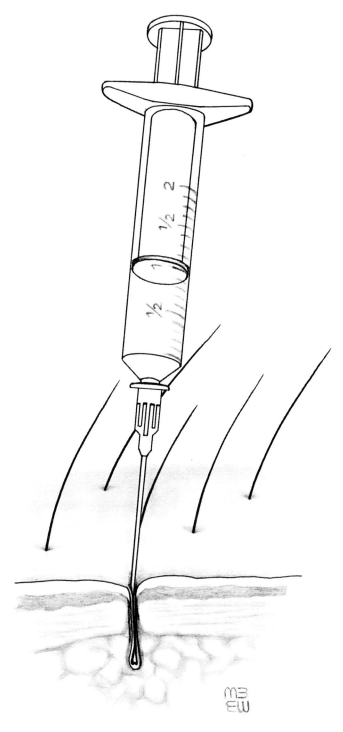

Fig 1. **Needle is inserted into an infundibular follicular structure to a plane above the perichondrium and below the dermis.**

REGIONAL ANESTHESIA FOR FACIAL COLLAGEN INJECTION

By Thomas Kohn, M.D.

Injection of collagen in the perioral area may be facilitated by a nerve block of both the upper and lower lips.

TECHNIQUE

The infraorbital nerve is blocked in a painless manner by the initial application of a topical anesthetic, such as 20% benzocaine, to the mucus membrane at the gumline at the level of the second premolar tooth. A 1- to 3-ml amount of 1% Xylocaine with epinephrine (Astra) is subsequently injected at the level of the second premolar in the direction of the midpupillary line. The overlying skin is subsequently massaged to distribute the anesthetic agent around the vicinity of the nerve. When the lip becomes heavy and anesthetic, collagen may be injected painlessly (Fig 1).

The mental nerve may be blocked in a similar fashion. The 20% benzocaine is applied topically to the mucus membrane in the vicinity of the second bicuspid tooth. A 1- to 3-ml amount of 1% Xylocaine with epinephrine is then injected through the anesthetized mucus membrane in the midpupillary line. To achieve full anesthesia of the lower lip, the procedure may need to be repeated once or twice.

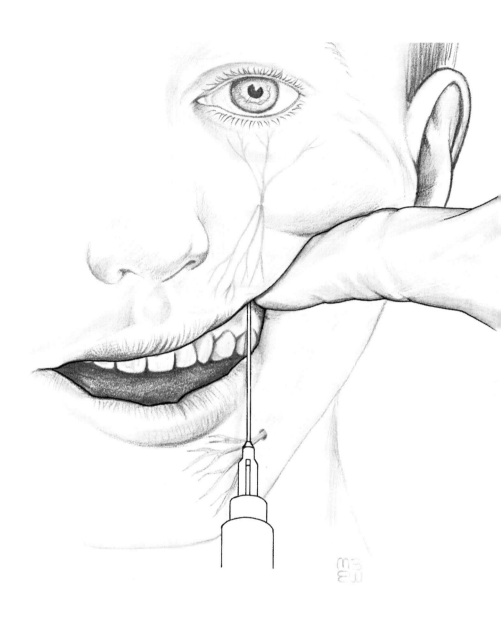

Fig 1. **Block of infraorbital nerve for collagen injection.**

REGIONAL BLOCK ANESTHESIA OF THE EAR

By Ronald G. Wheeland, M.D.

The greater auricular nerve arises from the second and third cervical nerves and supplies the posterior portion of the lateral surface of the auricle and a major portion of the medial surface of the ear.

TECHNIQUE

The nerve can be blocked by using a 0.5-in 30-gauge needle inserted at the junction of the earlobe with the skin of the neck, directly perpendicular to the full depth or hub of the needle (Fig 1). A 2-ml amount of 1% Xylocaine (Astra) is injected into this area and will provide anesthesia of the posterior and medial surface of the ear for up to 2 hr. This has the additional benefit of minimizing distortion of the helix and other anatomic landmarks of the ear, permitting precise localization of residual malignancies when performing Mohs micrographic surgery. Additional anesthesia can be achieved by a field block of the ear with injections superiorly and posteriorly as indicated in Figure 2.

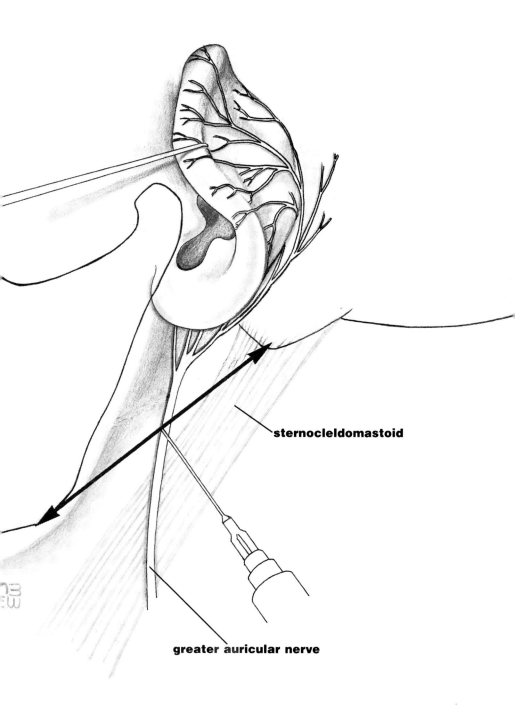

sternocleidomastoid

greater auricular nerve

Fig 1. **Technique for blocking greater auricular nerve.**

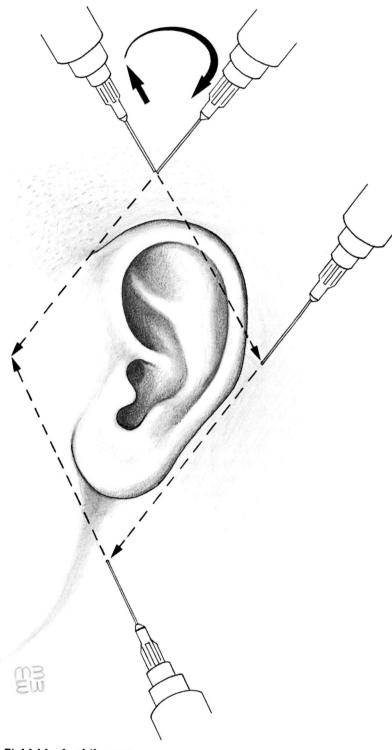

Fig 2.   **Field block of the ear.**

PART II

BIOPSIES, EXCISIONS, AND GENERAL DERMATOLOGIC PROCEDURES

BIOPSY OF ORAL LESIONS

By Roger I. Ceilley, M.D.,
and Eugene L. Bodian, M.D.

Biopsy of lesions of oral mucosa is complicated by poor visibility, mucosal mobility, excessive bleeding, and difficulties with closure. Two special techniques can be used to simplify biopsy.[1]

TECHNIQUES

A) The mucosal surface is dried with gauze. Gentian violet is used to mark out the lesion. Local anesthetic is infiltrated with a 30-gauge needle. A chalazion clamp is positioned with the open ring of the clamp surrounding the lesion. The screw is tightened until it fits snugly in order to produce immobility and hemostasis. The biopsy is performed within the confines of the clamp ring (Fig 1). Sutures are best inserted prior to release of the clamp. This technique can greatly simplify mucosal biopsy and can be used in a similar fashion for tongue biopsies.

B) Preliminary sutures can be placed around an oral mucosal lesion prior to excision. This technique allows immobilization of the mucosa with the suture. The lesion is excised, and the defect is closed with the suture (Figs 2 to 4). Putting in sutures before biopsy allows rapid control of bleeding, as the sutures are already in place and can be easily tied to control hemostasis.

REFERENCE
1. Ceilley R. Surgical gems: Biopsy technique for oral lesions. J Dermatol Surg Oncol 5:88–89, 1979.

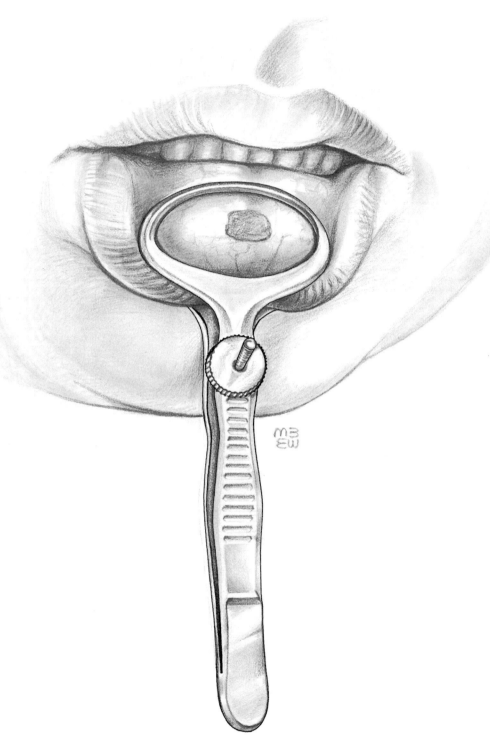

Fig 1. **Chalazion clamp in place over an oral lesion.**

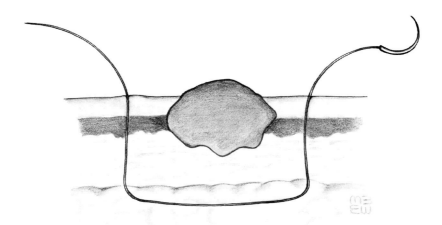

Fig 2.   **Suture before excision.**

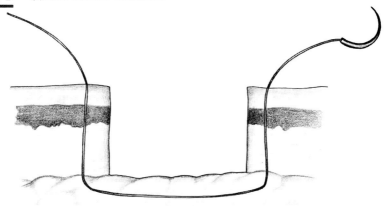

Fig 3.   **Excision, showing margin and suture.**

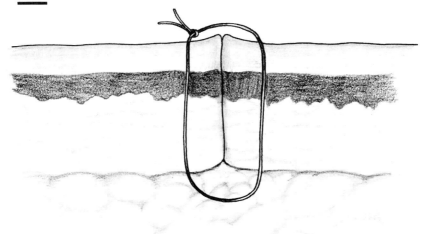

Fig 4.   **Closure of defect.**

CURETTAGE FOLLOWED BY EXCISIONAL SURGERY

By Perry Robins, M.D., and Russell W. Cohen, M.D.

The curette is one of the most useful surgical instruments available to the dermatologist. Based on its ability to differentiate between diseased and normal tissue, the curette has been used to treat a variety of benign and malignant lesions. As far as the treatment of basal cell and squamous cell carcinomas is concerned, most dermatologists are skeptical about the use of curettage alone. Over the past years, other destructive modalities have been combined with curettage. These include the use of radiation, electrodesiccation or electrocoagulation, and liquid nitrogen.[1]

The goal in the treatment of basal cell and squamous cell carcinomas is complete removal of the tumor with the best possible cosmetic result. Of the standard methods for treatment of these skin carcinomas, excisional surgery will usually attain both goals. However, excisional surgery relies on the visual delineation of the extent of involvement of the tumor, and therefore must include an approximate amount of normal-appearing tissue to ensure the entire tumor will be destroyed. Recommended margins range from 2 to 10 mm.

Curettage for peripheral spread and depth of a biopsy-proven basal cell or squamous cell carcinoma followed by excisional surgery just beyond the curettage is an easy and effective way of removing the tumor without relying on visual estimation of subclinical invasion. This combined method provides two benefits to the dermatologic surgeon. First, because a significant amount of normal tissue is spared, the size of the excision may be decreased and hence a more cosmetically acceptable result attained. Second, and more important, curettage may reveal lateral or deep extensions of the tumor that were not obvious clinically (Figs 1 to 3). This will prevent underestimation of the breadth and depth of the lesion, which may lead to a positive margin and the need for repeat excision with wider margins.

This combined method is not useful for all basal cell and squamous cell carcinomas. It is not recommended for skin carcinomas that require Mohs micrographic surgery. It is, however, an easy and effective method of treating classic basal cell and squamous cell carcinomas with a relatively high assurance of complete removal of the tumor with a significant sparing of normal tissue.

REFERENCE
1. Albright SD. Treatment of skin cancer using multiple modalities. J Am Acad Dermatol 7:143–171, 1982.

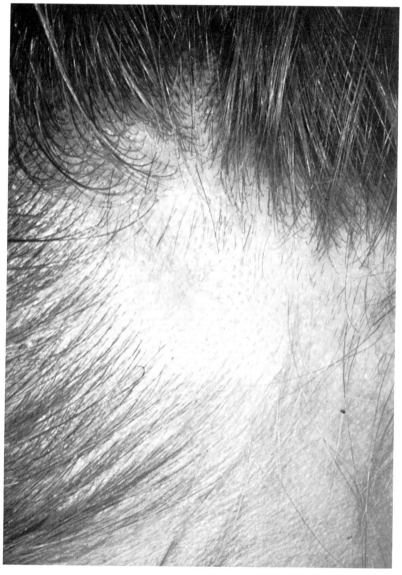

Fig 1   **Basal cell carcinoma with diffuse border preoperatively.**

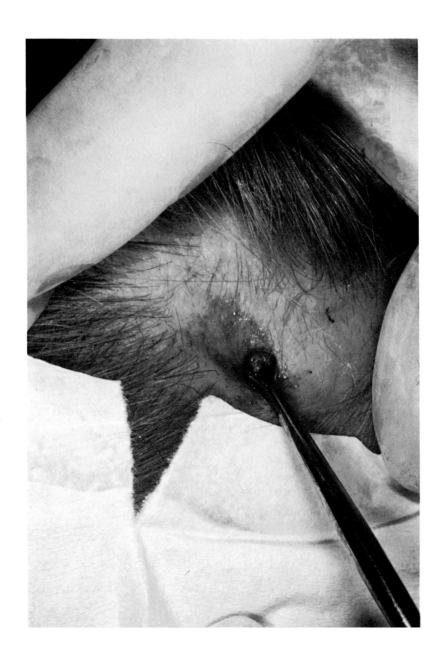

Fig 2.   Curettage reveals peripheral extension of the tumor.

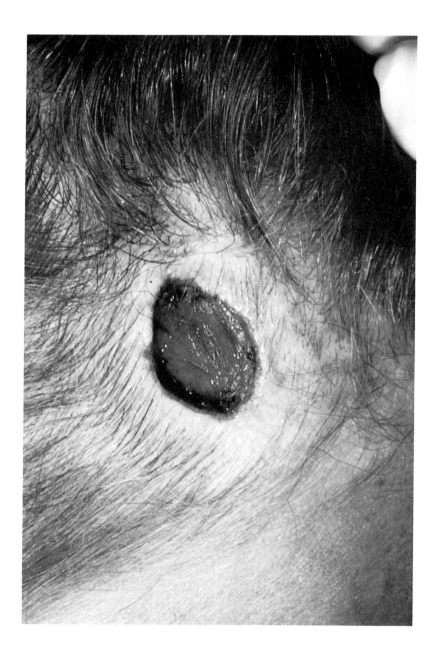

Fig 3.   **Final extent of involvement of tumor as approximated by
curettage.**

ESTIMATING THE MARGINS OF SCLEROTIC BASAL CELL CARCINOMA

By George R. Mikhail, M.D.

Estimating the clinical extent of a morpheic basal cell carcinoma is difficult. This accounts for the higher recurrence rate of this type of tumor with methods of treatment other than Mohs micrographic surgery. A simple examination technique can aid accurate definition of tumor margins.

TECHNIQUE

Stretching the skin firmly between thumb and index finger, as shown in the illustrations (Figs 1 and 2), demonstrates the translucent and waxy appearance of the edge of the tumor.

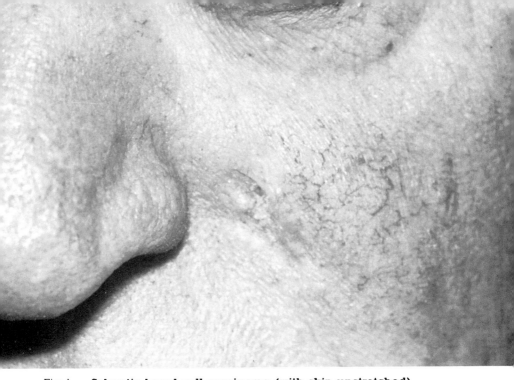

Fig 1.　Sclerotic basal cell carcinoma (with skin unstretched).

Fig 2.　Sclerotic basal cell carcinoma seen in Figure 1 with skin stretched.

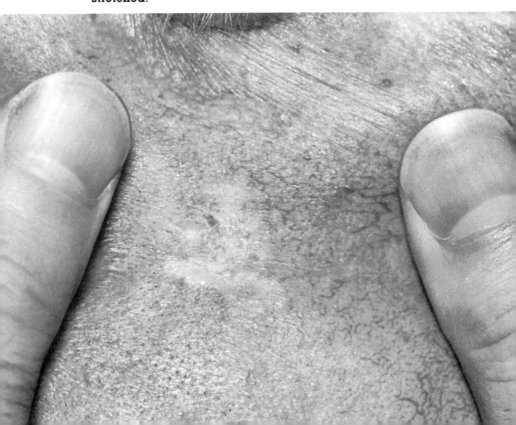

EXCISION OF BENIGN NEVI BY THE SHAVE TECHNIQUE IN AREAS OF THIN AND MOBILE SKIN

By Jean Arouete, M.D.

The shave excision technique is simple to perform where the skin is very thick, such as on the nose and face or on the back. However, in certain areas such as the dorsum of the hand, axilla, and abdomen, where the skin is thin and/or mobile, an inaccurate incision may be made because of lack of control of the scalpel blade.

TECHNIQUE

Local anesthetic is infiltrated into the base of the lesion, thereby producing a taut area of skin. The skin is grasped between thumb and forefinger with gauze if necessary, so as to tent up the lesion. A convex area is created around the surgeon's index finger. Because the area is now raised up and firm, it is simple to perform a precise shave excision (Fig 1).

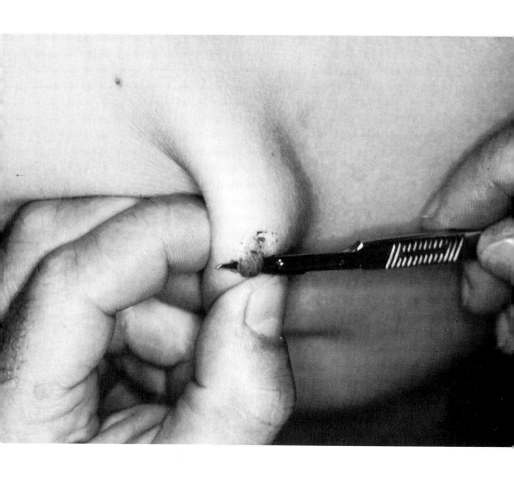

Fig 1. **Use of infiltration and the surgeon's finger to firm mobile skin for shave excision.**

MODIFIED M-PLASTY

By Saul Asken, M.D.

The original M-plasty developed to shorten the length of a scar was improved by Dr. Richard C. Webster. The creation of two triangular flaps at either end of the incision made possible a shorter scar, which can be further shortened by the use of the modified M-plasty procedure.

TECHNIQUE

The lesion is excised with a therapeutic margin in a circular, oval, or fusiform fashion without creating the initial triangular flap at either or both ends of the wound. Instead, an incision is then made parallel to the long axis of the wound, on either side, creating a triangular flap whose apex is on the "belly" of the wound, and whose base is at the level of the excision's tip (Fig 1). The newly created triangular flap is undermined and the apex of the flap is shifted toward the center of the wound, which is then closed in the usual manner. To avoid protrusion of the newly created triangular flap, it can be defatted and a suture can be passed through its dermis to assure its being level with the surrounding skin. There may be some protrusion at the pivot point of the flap, as it is rotated toward the center of the wound. This usually can be avoided by adequate undermining and the correct placement of sutures.

As can be seen in Figure 1, the modified M-plasty results in a significant shortening of the wound and the subsequent scar as compared with the routine fusiform excision as well as the traditional M-plasty. The modified M-plasty can be performed on one as well as on both apices of the wound. Furthermore, the triangular flaps can be created on the opposite sides of the excision, as illustrated in Figure 1, or on the same side of the wound, depending on its location. This procedure is useful wherever a shorter scar is preferred, particularly in facial surgery where the length of a traditional excision might encroach on important neighboring anatomic structures such as the eyelids.

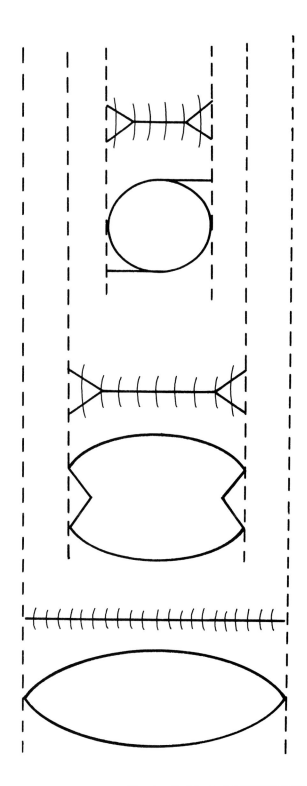

Fig 1. The standard fusiform incision, the traditional M-plasty, and the modified M-plasty with their respective closures.

REMOVAL OF INTRADERMAL NEVI AND SIMILAR BENIGN LESIONS

By Enrique Hernández-Pérez, M.D.

Most intradermal nevi and other similar benign lesions, such as trichoepithelioma and small cysts, are removed from the face for cosmetic reasons. It is imperative, therefore, that the resulting scar be as imperceptible as possible.

Traditionally, these small lesions have been handled by means of shaving and electrodesiccation or hemostasis with Monsel's solution. Although this method provides material for histopathology and permits partial destruction of the base, scarring has not always been as adequate as one would wish. In many instances, a better result can be achieved with the use of a punch biopsy.

TECHNIQUE

Following disinfection of an area and injection of 1% lidocaine with epinephrine, a punch is selected, the diameter of which should be slightly larger than the lesion to be excised. The skin is stretched between thumb and index fingers in the opposite direction to the natural wrinkle line, and the punch is advanced with a rapid twisting motion. Once the lesion is completely excised, the circular defect will tend to become ovoid in the direction of the natural skin wrinkle lines. Hemostasis is achieved by electrocautery. Following suture with 5-0 or 6-0 nylon, small dog ears occur at either end of the defect. These can be simply removed by elevating them with a skin hook and cutting with a single stroke using curved iris scissors (Fig 1).

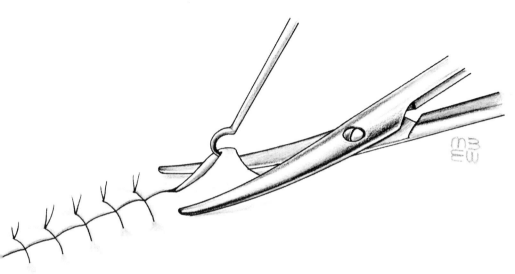

Fig 1. **Removal of dog ears with iris scissors.**

THE RHOMBIC FLAP

By Carl Vinciullo, M.B., B.S.

The rhombic flap is an extremely useful technique for the closure of relatively large defects. Design of the flap should produce a rhombus, i.e., an equilateral parallelogram with all sides of the defect and the rhombic flap of equal length, with the opposing angles consisting of either 60° or 120°. Analysis of the angles shows that if there were no differences in skin tension, it would be futile to use the rhombic flap. Closure of the defect left by the donor rhombic flap would be almost impossible. In clinical practice with poorly designed rhombic flaps, it is in fact closure of the secondary defect that is most frequently the cause of problems. For this reason, some basic principles must be applied in designing the flap to avoid these problems.[1]

TECHNIQUE

The short diagonal of the donor area of the rhombic flap should fall exactly in the direction of the lines of maximal extensibility. To achieve this, the first step in designing the flap should be to draw parallel lines following the lines of maximal extensibility (at right angles to the relaxed skin tension, or wrinkle lines).

Two other lines are drawn to complete the design of an equilateral parallelogram with 60° or 120° angles. The lesion should be included within the design of the rhombus, with the least amount of sacrifice of normal tissue, yet with a safe margin of tissue around the lesion. The next step is to draw a line as an extension of the short diagonal of the rhombic defect, with the other legs parallel to one of its sides. All sides of the defect and the rhombic flap are of equal length with opposing angles of 60° and 120°, but this still leaves four possible rhombic flaps to choose from, two on either side of the defect.

Deciding which of the four flaps to use is determined by identifying the flap in which the short diagonal follows the line of maximal extensibility. A simple clinical way to test this is to "pinch" each of the V's created by the rhombic flap design. The V in which there is maximal mobility of skin will be the flap that follows the line of maximal extensibility (Fig 1).

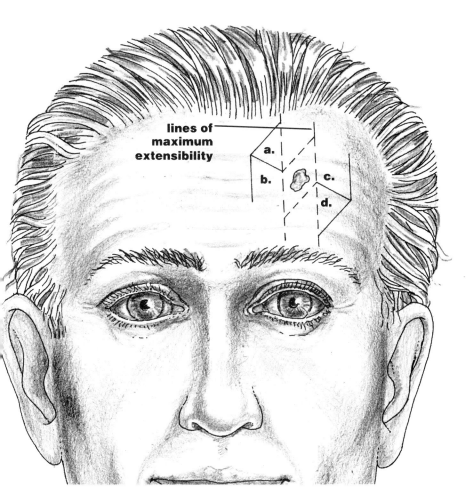

lines of maximum extensibility

a.

b.

c.

d.

Fig 1. **Of the four possible rhombic flaps drawn, only (a) and (d) have their short diagonals parallel to the lines of maximum extensibility and therefore will allow closure of the secondary defect with relatively little tension.**

Additionally, consideration must be given to normal anatomic landmarks in choosing which rhombic flap to use. If the appropriate flap using geometric calculation will result in a distortion of anatomic landmarks, then one must consider using an alternative type of flap.

Notwithstanding the attractive geometry of the flap, the skin is not a geometric organ. Therefore, although these rules may be used for guidelines, they should not be adhered to absolutely to the exclusion of clinical judgment.

REFERENCE
1. Borges AF. The rhombic flap. Plast Reconstruct Surg 67:458–466, 1981.

SURGICAL MANAGEMENT OF HYPERHIDROSIS

By Annalis Scherrer-Koch, M.D.

There exists a simple surgical treatment for the common disorder of hyperhidrosis axillaris. This surgery can be performed on an outpatient basis under local anesthesia in approximately 45 min per side.

TECHNIQUE

Satisfactory results depend on excision of an area wider than the zone of most intense perspiration defined by Minor's perspiration test. The area of excision is marked with gentian violet on the fusiform, hair-bearing area of the axilla and subsequently injected with 30 ml of 0.5% lidocaine with epinephrine (1:200,000) or, alternatively, with POR 8 (Sandoz) for both anesthesia and marked vasoconstriction of the entire surgical site (Fig 1).

The axillary skin is excised at the level of the upper part of the subcutaneous fatty tissue, as shown in Figure 2. The wound edges are approximated by use of 2-0 Dexon sutures (Davis & Geck) subcutaneously buried and 4-0 Dexon sutures cutaneously (Fig 3). Other suture materials can be used, but nylon should be avoided, as this product may result in stiff, sharp suture ends, which the patient may find uncomfortable.

A gauze dressing is applied, and the upper arm is immobilized by elastic bandages, strapping the arm to the anterior chest.

For the next 5 postoperative days, the patient returns daily for a change in dressing. After 1 week, the upper arm no longer needs to be immobilized. The stitches are removed on postoperative day 12. After 20 days, the patient has usually recovered full mobility and can return to work. Of course, if both axillae are operated on at one session, it is necessary for the patient to have someone at home to provide care.

With full mobilization, the scar turns livid, but cosmetic results are quite satisfactory at 1 year. Movement is not restricted if the patient follows instructions.

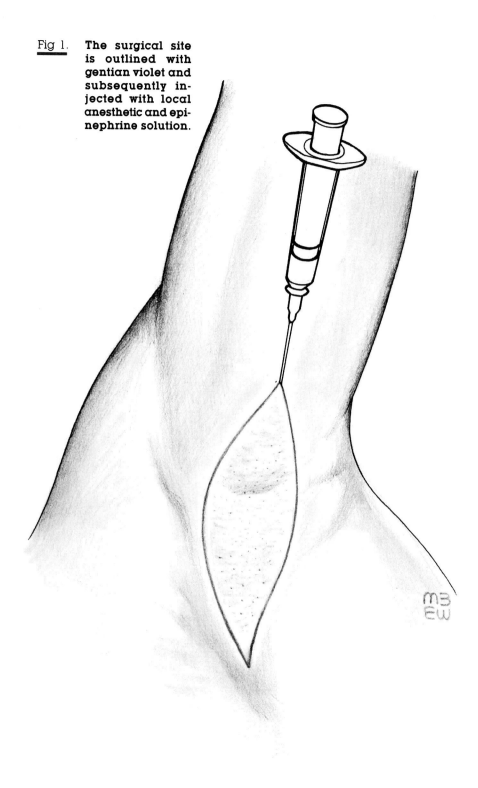

Fig 1. The surgical site is outlined with gentian violet and subsequently injected with local anesthetic and epinephrine solution.

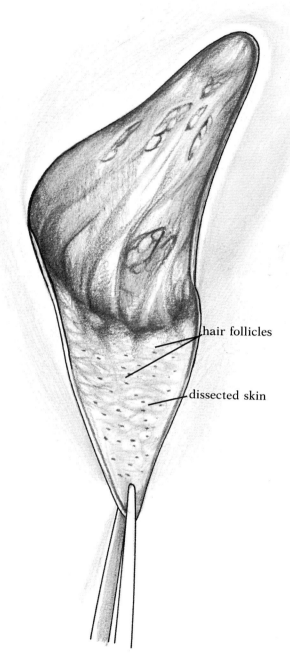

hair follicles

dissected skin

Fig 2. **Surgical site, showing skin dissected.**

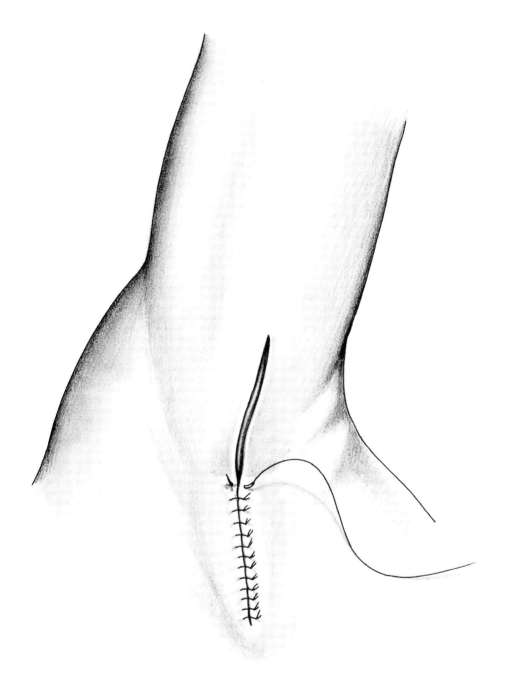

Fig 3.   **Wound closure.**

TREATMENT OF EPIDERMAL CYSTS

By Rafael Falabella, M.D.

Complete surgical removal of large epidermal inclusion cysts on the face can produce a significant area of scarring.

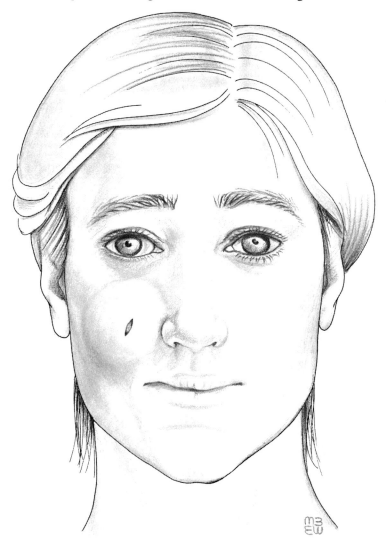

Fig 1a. **Drainage of epidermal cyst.**

TECHNIQUE

A small incision a few millimeters long into the cyst will permit drainage and reduction in size of the cyst (Fig 1a). Definitive excision is carried out 4 to 8 weeks later, with a resultant smaller wound and scar (Fig 1b).

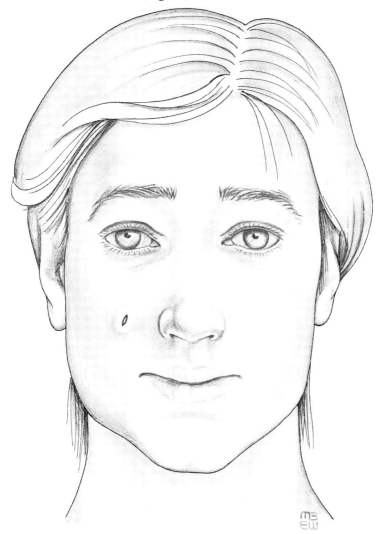

Fig 1b. **Smaller wound and scar.**

TREATMENT OF GRANULATION TISSUE BY CURETTAGE

By Blas A. Reyes, M.D., and Perry Robins, M.D.

Granulation tissue consists of multiple thin blood vessels in an edematous stroma containing fibroblasts and a mixed cellular infiltrate, which is the initial body response toward self-repair. The granulation process continues until it fills the defect. Mechanisms exist that control the formation of granulation tissue.

In some clinical situations, these mechanisms fail and granulation continues, resulting in an exophytic friable tissue. This hypergranulation interferes with the normal healing process and increases the risk of complications, such as bleeding and infection, which is frequently seen in surgical wounds allowed to heal by second intention.

TECHNIQUE

Classic management of this excessive granulation tissue consists of application of silver nitrate to these sites. Another method that is highly effective is gentle curettage of the hypergranulation tissue until one senses the presence of healthy fibrous tissue; a 3, 4, or 5 curette is used in a similar fashion to the curettage done for the treatment of basal cell carcinomas (Figs 1 to 3). Local anesthesia is not necessary, and the procedure can be performed with little or no pain. Some bleeding will occur on completion of the process, but firm pressure for a short time will provide adequate hemostasis. Once we have treated the wound we allow the healing process to begin again, hoping that the mechanisms controlling the growth of granulation will work properly. A few patients have a recurrence of excessive granulation tissue, indicating an intrinsic defect in the patient's healing mechanism. The same method may be repeated as many times as necessary; each time the area becomes smaller until it is finally healed.

This is a fast, simple method of treatment for hypergranulation tissue. It offers the advantage of removing all granulation tissue at once, while silver nitrate only removes the superficial layers. It also avoids the risk of localized argyria.

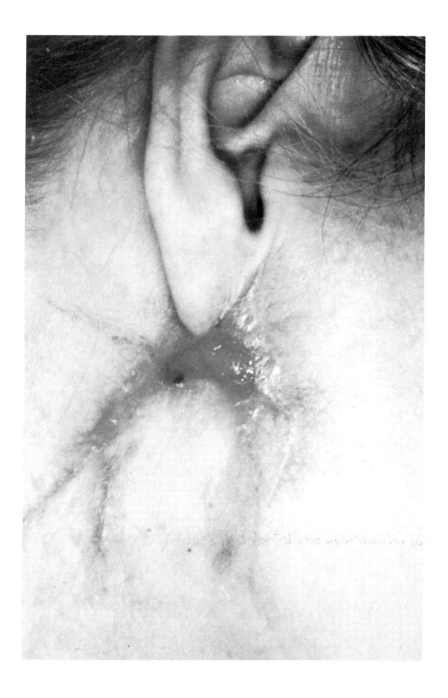

Fig 1.   **Excessive granulation tissue following partial necrosis of flap.**

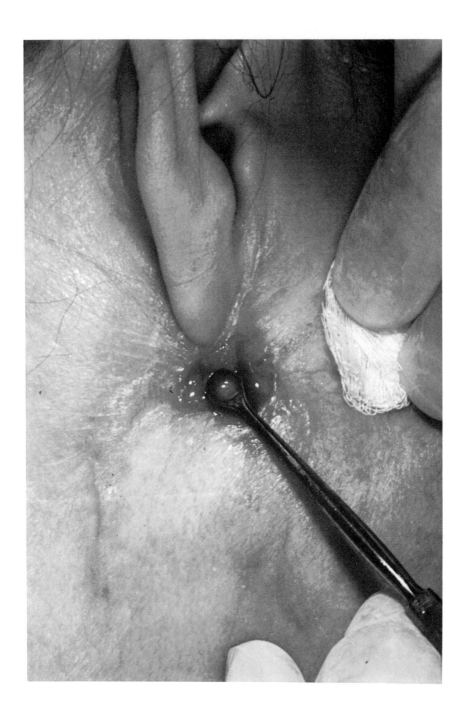

Fig 2.   Granulation tissue is curetted gently until one senses the presence of healthy fibrous tissue.

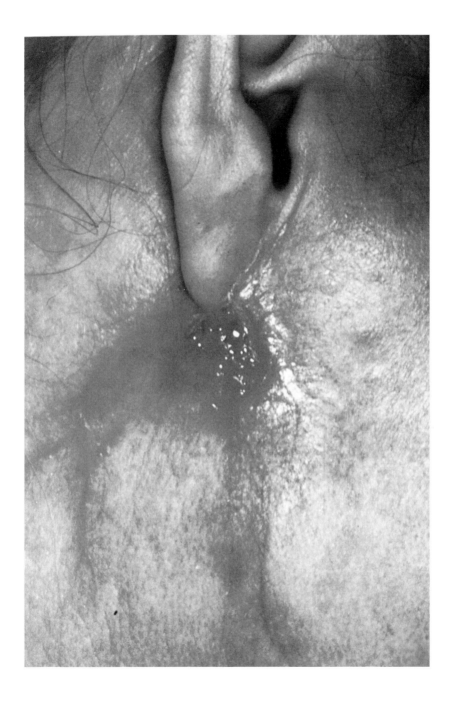

<u>Fig 3.</u> After completion of the curettage, bleeding is stopped by firm
pressure. The area is then allowed to start the healing process
once again.

PART III

DERMABRASION

DERMABRASION OF HANDS

By Ervin Epstein, M.D.

Dermabrasion of the dorsa of the hands offers protection against the subsequent development of keratoses and epitheliomas as well as the safe elimination of the alterations produced by chronic solar irradiation.

In the experience of this dermatologist, only a few patients who have undergone this procedure have subsequently developed an occasional keratosis, and none have developed an epithelioma. In this respect, dermabrasion may be superior to applications of 5-fluorouracil.

Because the skin is very thin in this area, especially in older patients, special caution is necessary, since large blood vessels, nerves, and tendons lie just beneath the surface. The ballooning out of the skin by subcutaneous injection of local anesthetic is the key to success (Fig 1). This procedure eliminates the necessity of freezing the skin and allows planing of the skin to be done easily, rapidly, and safely. The author's personal preference is for a Dremel Hand Tool (Dremel) with a rheostat to control the speed of rotation. However, any of the available alternative hand engines will serve the same purpose. A diamond fraize is preferred over a wirebrush, as this is more controllable. The wirebrush may easily produce severe gouging and cause damage to the underlying structures. With reasonable care, one can eliminate keratoses and epitheliomas quickly and easily. Also, the skin of the dorsum of the hand has a well-deserved reputation for healing with minimal scarring.

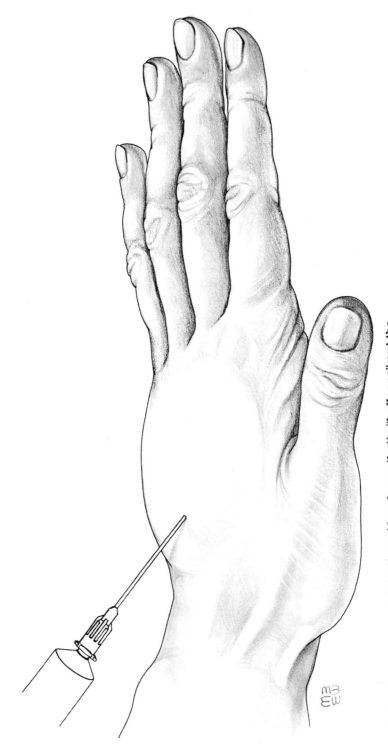

Fig 1. Subcutaneous injection of local anesthetic "balloons" out the skin prior to dermabrasion of the dorsum of the hand and eliminates the need for freezing.

PUNCH FLOAT TECHNIQUE FOR "ICE-PICK" SCARS

By John M. Yarborough, Jr., M.D., and Edward F. Pitard, M.D.

The punch float technique can be used to complement dermabrasion for the acne-scarred face. The technique is very useful for those "ice-pick" scars usually unreachable by dermabrasion.

TECHNIQUE

Each pit is first marked with gentian violet using the blunt end of a cotton-tipped swab. Local anesthetic is then injected into the area. The usual size of these lesions varies from 1 to 4 mm in diameter, and we then use a punch just large enough to fill the defect while the skin is stretched. The punch is driven to the level of subcutaneous fat (Fig 1). Pressure is then applied to the sides of the incision with the thumbs or fingers. The graft usually "floats" to the surface (Fig 2). Occasionally gentle coaxing with micro-Adson forceps is necessary. The floated graft is allowed to sit for a few minutes, until the coagulum is sticky enough to hold the graft in place. Vigilon (Hermal) is then applied for 2 days. The area usually heals with a smoother surface, and dermabrasion can then be performed in 4 to 6 weeks.

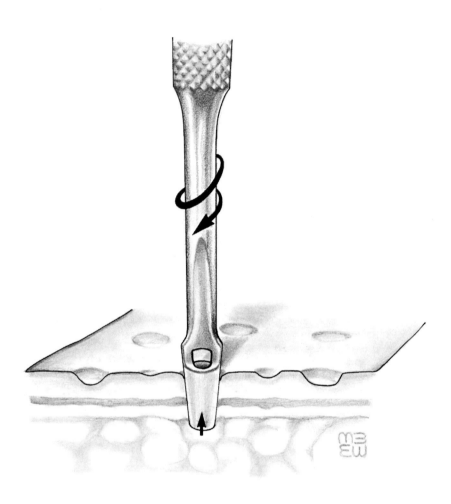

Fig 1. Punch being driven to level of subcutaneous fat.

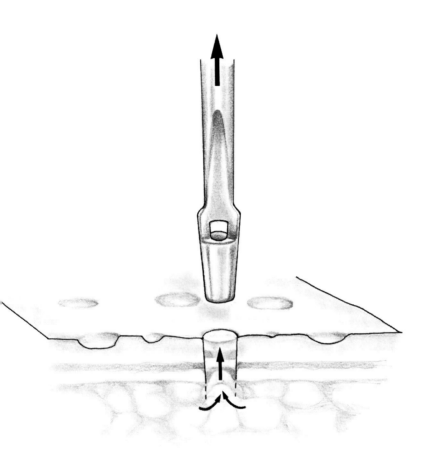

Fig 2.　Graft "floating" to skin surface.

VIGILON AS A DERMABRASION DRESSING

By John L. Ratz, M.D.

Postoperative discomfort is one of the greatest problems following facial dermabrasion. This can be substantially reduced and even eliminated by using the following techniques.

TECHNIQUE

Following completion of dermabrasion, the area is gently cleaned with a solution of chlorhexidine gluconate (Hibiclens, Stuart). Following this, an antibacterial ointment can be applied to the dermabraded area. A strip of Vigilon (Hermal) is taken, and the polyethylene is removed from one side. The Vigilon is placed gel side down over the dermabraded area. A bulky dressing is then placed over the Vigilon, and the patient asked to return 24 hr later. At that point, the dressing is removed and replaced with a similar one. Subsequently, the patient is able to remove the dressing without discomfort and begin a gentle cleansing program using chlorhexidine gluconate followed by antibacterial ointment. This may be repeated several times daily until re-epithelialization is complete. Vigilon, an inert dressing composed of 4% polyethylene oxide and 96% water in a colloidal suspension sandwiched between two polyethylene films, has been shown to enhance re-epithelialization. By providing a moist environment for wound healing, it diminishes pain as well.

PART IV

SURGICAL PROCEDURES OF THE EAR

Cryosurgery of Malignancies on the Ear
By Emanuel G. Kuflik, M.D.

Facial Scar Revision with Full-Thickness Autologous Punch
Grafting from the Posterior Earlobe
By David S. Orentreich, M.D., and Norman Orentreich, M.D.

Harvesting of the Earlobe and Helical Reconstruction
By Jeffrey H. Binstock, M.D.

Punch Excisions Through the Cartilage for Ear Defects
By Perry Robins, M.D.

CRYOSURGERY OF MALIGNANCIES ON THE EAR

By Emanuel G. Kuflik, M.D.

Cryosurgery of malignancies on the ear can lead to cartilage necrosis if an excessive depth of freeze is achieved.

TECHNIQUE

Anesthetic can be injected locally in the perichondrial plane to lift the tumor away from the underlying cartilage. This is possible only if the tumor has not penetrated deep to the perichondrium. The "ballooning" enables the operator to freeze the tumor adequately and to ensure eradication without risking cartilage necrosis.

FACIAL SCAR REVISION WITH FULL-THICKNESS AUTOLOGOUS PUNCH GRAFTING FROM THE POSTERIOR EARLOBE

By David S. Orentreich, M.D., and Norman Orentreich, M.D.

The objective of cutaneous rehabilitative surgery is to impart a more acceptable physical appearance to the surface of the skin. Although a total correction of the tissue deformities caused by acne and other scarring dermatoses cannot always be achieved, the rationale for such surgery goes beyond the cosmetic to a concern for improving the patient's self-image.

A scar can be characterized as narrow or wide, deep or shallow, pitted, "ice-pick"-like, "crater"-like, diffusely depressed, hypotrophic, hypertrophic, keloidal, hypopigmented, or hyperpigmented. Rehabilitation techniques are tailored to the type of scar (Fig 1). The typical acne patient has a variety of scar types, and several different techniques usually are required to achieve optimal reconstruction.[1] It is advisable to have good preoperative and postoperative photographic documentation.

PUNCH ELEVATION

A depressed scar with normal surface texture may be improved simply by punch elevation with a cylindrical biopsy punch (Fig 2). The depressed area is raised to a level flush with the surrounding skin. Occasionally, suturing may be needed to secure the graft in its elevated position during healing;[2] it may be necessary to desiccate the edges after healing. Apart from acne, other scarring conditions can be treated in a similar fashion: smallpox, chickenpox, herpes zoster, and rarer conditions such as necrotic tuberculids.[3] Similarly, one can correct scars resulting from the excision or destruction of small cutaneous tumors.[4]

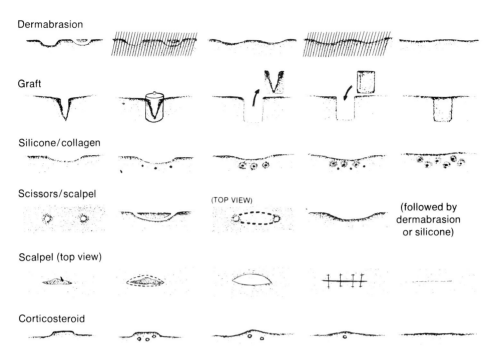

Dermabrasion

Graft

Silicone/collagen

Scissors/scalpel

(TOP VIEW)

(followed by dermabrasion or silicone)

Scalpel (top view)

Corticosteroid

Fig 1. Treatments for multiform acne scars. A variety of treatments may be required for optimal improvement. Dermabrasion smoothes sharp-edged scars and breaks up fibrotic bases. Free full-thickness earlobe skin grafts replace deep, patulous, epithelialized infundibular tracts. Silicone droplets at the appropriate depth stimulate collagen augmentation of depressed scars.* Either dermabrasion or excision unroofs epithelialized sinuses. Large confluent areas of scarring may by excised and sutured. Intralesional injections of corticosteroids intentionally atrophy hypertrophic and keloidal scars. (Reprinted from Dermatologic Clinics, Vol 5, No 2: Advanced Dermatologic Surgery. Philadelphia, WB Saunders, 1987, p 360.)

*Orentreich DS, Orentreich N. Injectable fluid silicone. In Roenigk RK, Roenigk HH (eds): Principles of Dermatologic Surgery. New York, Marcel Dekker. In press.

PUNCH EXCISION WITH FULL-THICKNESS AUTOLOGOUS PUNCH GRAFT REPLACEMENT

Although punch elevation is helpful in treating scars of depressed but otherwise normal skin, punch excision with immediate full-thickness grafting is more often needed for optimal cosmetic results.

Punch excision surgery with graft replacement is suited for patients either with a few discrete acne scars or with scars not amenable to improvement by dermabrasion and/or silicone or

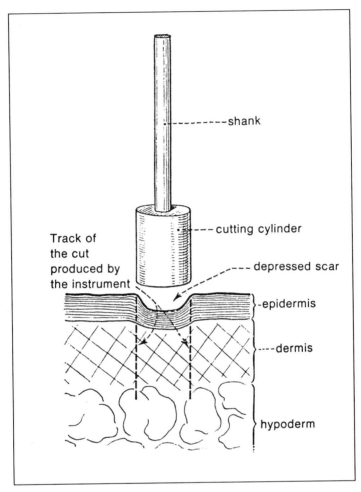

Fig 2. **Schema of incision of the skin by means of a punch for elevation of scars.**

collagen augmentation. The ideal scar for punch excision and grafting is the "ice-pick" scar, which is, essentially, an epithelial tract in which bands of collagen fix the epithelial invagination to the subcutaneous layer. When keratin, sebaceous, and bacterial debris collect in these epithelialized invaginations with resultant episodic inflammatory responses, they become epithelialized infundibular cysts.

Additional skin lesions amenable to the autologous punch grafting method of rehabilitation include trichostasis spinulosa, isolated large pores, giant comedones, small epidermoid cysts and steatocystomas, nevi, and those scarring conditions treatable by punch elevation.

TECHNIQUE

The donor (posterior earlobe) and recipient (defect) sites are locally anesthetized with 1% lidocaine, usually containing epinephrine 1:100,000. The defect is excised with a biopsy punch, typically 2 to 3 mm in diameter, and submitted for histopathologic examination or discarded (Fig 1). We prefer the Orentreich punch (Robbins Instruments), a cylindrical metal punch with a knurled handle and a hole in the cylinder for easy cleaning (Fig 3). A graft of normal skin is punch excised from the posterior earlobe. Because of the elastic recoil property of the skin, the recipient site spreads and the donor skin graft shrinks; therefore, the donor skin graft usually is excised with a punch slightly larger (25% to 50%) than the one used to excise the defect, assuring a snug fit. Trimming of fat from the donor graft or suturing of either site is rarely needed.

If the patient is a male and the recipient site is within his beard area, then the posterior hair-bearing scalp is used for the donor site, and some trimming of the graft's subcutaneous tissue may be required. However, care is taken to avoid inadvertent trimming of the dermal papillae.

If the defect is elliptical, it can be excised with a circular punch by stretching the defect across its short axis, thereby creating a circular defect. The donor tissue is also excised in a similar manner, with one axis stretched to produce an elliptical graft.

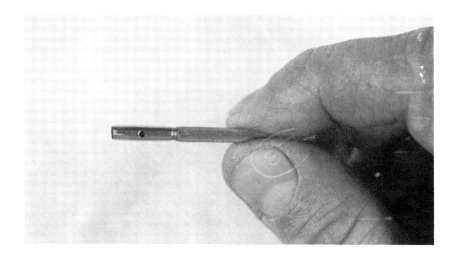

Fig 3.   **The Orentreich punch.**

Multiple autologous punch grafts may be performed conveniently in a single office visit. Ordinarily, the maximal number is ten per session, and these may all be harvested from one healthy earlobe. Certain patients with a history of severe acne may have earlobes that are so cystic and scarred they are inappropriate donor sites. In these patients, the postauricular skin or the proximal, medial, or upper arm skin may be used.

After the donor graft is placed and hemostasis is achieved by firm pressure, each graft is covered with a 3M Micropore skintone surgical tape dressing. Hemostasis at the recipient and donor sites is achieved with manual pressure instead of such hemostatic agents as ferric subsulfate (Monsel's solution) or aluminum chloride that may interfere with healing and graft survival by delaying vascularization.

The tape dressing is left in place to protect the graft for 5 days. The patient is advised to apply direct firm pressure if bleeding occurs from either site after leaving the doctor's office. Makeup may be applied over the tape or after the tape has been removed, but the makeup should be removed gently. After removing the dressing, an antibiotic ointment is applied sparingly to the donor and recipient sites several times a day for about 3 more days to prevent desiccation necrosis. The surgical sites may be gently washed so long as contact with irritating soaps or chemicals is avoided.

Before leaving the office, the patient is given instructions to follow if a graft comes out:

1) Handle it very gently, and cleanse it in an 8-ounce glass of tepid water to which ¼ teaspoon of salt has been added.
2) Wrap it in a clean handkerchief saturated with some of the mildly salted water.
3) Store the wet-wrapped graft in the refrigerator (not the freezer) for no more than 4 days.
4) Call the office for an appointment the same or next day to have the graft replaced. If the graft is lost or cannot be saved, the site can always be regrafted.

For optimal cosmetic results, a fully healed graft may need leveling by electrodesiccation or tangential excision 4 weeks or more after grafting. If the patient has extensive and varied scarring (as from acne), which is suitable for grafting and dermabrasion, then dermabrasion is usually done after grafting in order to also blend the grafts. If a graft heals significantly lower than the surrounding skin, the site may be treated by silicone or collagen augmentation, punch elevation, or reexcision and replacement with a slightly larger punch graft. Color discrepancy, if any, between the sun-protected grafted tissue and the surrounding sun-exposed facial skin usually resolves within 3 months. During this lag period, patients are instructed to protect the grafted skin from undue sun exposure by application of a sunscreen.

Autologous punch grafting has several advantages over other methods of excision: incapacitation, residual tissue defect, and cosmetic inconvenience are minimized during the healing period.

REFERENCES
1. Orentreich DS, Orentreich N. Acne scar revision update. In Balin PL, Ratz JL, Wheeland RG (eds): Dermatologic Clinics, Vol 5, No 2: Advanced Dermatologic Surgery. Philadelphia, WB Saunders, 1987, pp 359–368.
2. Orentreich N, Orentreich DS. "Cross-stitch" suture technique for hair transplantation. J Dermatol Surg Oncol 10:970–971, 1984.
3. Arouete J. Correction of depressed scars on the face by a method of elevation. J Dermatol Surg Oncol 2:337–339, 1976.
4. Deutsch HL, Orentreich N. Treatment of small external cancers of the nose. Ann Plast Surg 3:567–571, 1979.

HARVESTING OF THE EARLOBE AND HELICAL RECONSTRUCTION

By Jeffrey H. Binstock, M.D.

Resection of skin cancers overlying the helical rim frequently results in a through-and-through defect because the tumor has spread perichondrially, with extension over both the anterior and posterior surfaces of the helical cartilage. Such defects vary in size and shape and challenge the skill of those who seek to restore helical integrity. The defects may involve the helical rim alone or may extend to the anthelix and even the concha.

TECHNIQUES

Chondrocutaneous advancement and/or rotation flaps are readily accomplished provided the defect lies over the superior two-thirds of the ear and does not represent a greater than 40% loss of the ear. The problem is twofold: a helical rim, or edge, must be created; and the defect, if present in the anthelix or concha, must be closed.

The earlobe serves as a reservoir of skin that will allow advancement and/or rotation of the entire remaining helix up-wards. As seen in Figure 1, this flap can be created by incising the helical rim through and through and extending the incision into the earlobe. It is also possible to incise the anterior skin and cartilage, almost severing the earlobe anteriorly, while retaining posterior skin that has been freed to the postauricular sulcus. This maneuver creates a rotation-and-advancement flap that al-lows significant movement of the helix, but only if the flap has been extended into the earlobe. When the defect is of the helical rim without involving the body of the ear, that is, the anthelix and concha, this is often all that is necessary to effect closure.

If the defect extends into the anthelix with or without in-volvement of the concha, then this maneuver will not only enclose the rim, but also help to increase the vertical height of the reconstructed ear. Wedges, triangles of skin and cartilage, can be removed from the anthelix and concha to enable these structures to collapse as they rotate together (Figs 2 and 3). If a substantial area of the anthelix and concha is involved, the cartilage and skin wedges that are removed can be used as composite grafts to rebuild within the remaining defect in the anthelix and concha. Again, this helps to increase the end height of the reconstructed ear.

In summary, harvesting the earlobe facilitates the closure of helical rim defects and, when necessary, can be combined with wedge resection of the anterior anthelix with or without the concha to effect closure of large defects. The wedges of skin and cartilage removed from the anthelix and concha can be used in turn as composite grafts to effect closure.

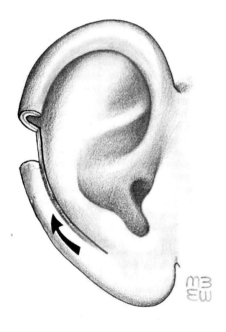
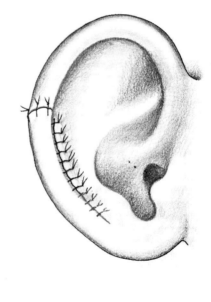

Fig 1.   **A flap is created by incising the helical rim through and through and extending into the earlobe.**

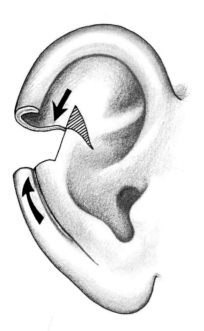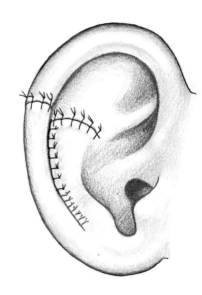

Fig 2. **Wedges removed from the skin and cartilage allow closure of a defect of rim and anthelix (and concha).**

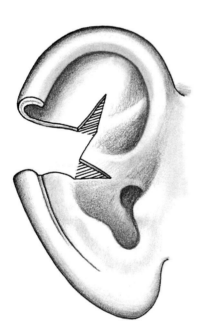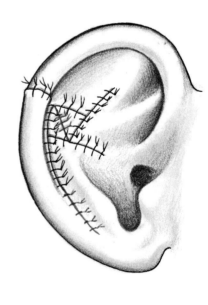

Fig 3. **The "triangles" removed from the anthelix and concha allow these structures to collapse as they rotate together. Skin and cartilage triangle-shaped wedges serve as composite grafts to close large defects.**

PUNCH EXCISIONS THROUGH THE CARTILAGE FOR EAR DEFECTS

By Perry Robins, M.D.

Surgical defects of the ear may be difficult to correct. Multiple flaps and grafts have been designed for reconstruction.[1] Healing of defects by second intention occasionally provides acceptable cosmetic results. However, we may be confronted with a defect so large that healing is not possible, increasing the risk of loss of the cartilaginous framework. In cases in which the perichondrium has been removed, split-thickness grafts are not a good alternative since they often will not survive without the presence of a vascular base.

A simple, effective, and rapid method to promote the growth of granulation tissue is presented. Multiple small 1- to 3-mm punch excisions are made through the cartilage to remove it, with care taken not to perforate the dermis on the other side (Figs 1 to 3). This can be accomplished easily without anesthesia, with only minimal discomfort.

The granulation tissue will progress, not only from the borders of the defect, but also through the passages within the cartilage, decreasing the granulation time. Once granulation tissue has covered the defect, a split-thickness graft may be placed with an increased chance of success or the wound may be seen to re-epithelialize at a faster rate. The cartilage must be protected from air-drying at all times.

This procedure was first presented at a Mohs surgery conference in 1965 by John F. Latenser, M.D., of Omaha, Nebraska.

REFERENCE
1. Converse JM, Brent B. Acquired deformities of the auricle. In Converse JM, et al (eds): Reconstructive Plastic Surgery. Philadelphia, WB Saunders, 1977, p 571.

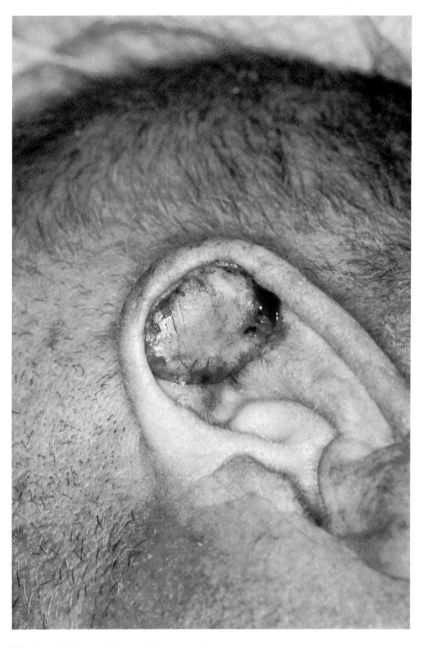

Fig 1.   A large 3.5 × 2.8-cm defect involving scaphoid fossa and anthelix. (Courtesy of Dr. Roy Geronemus.)

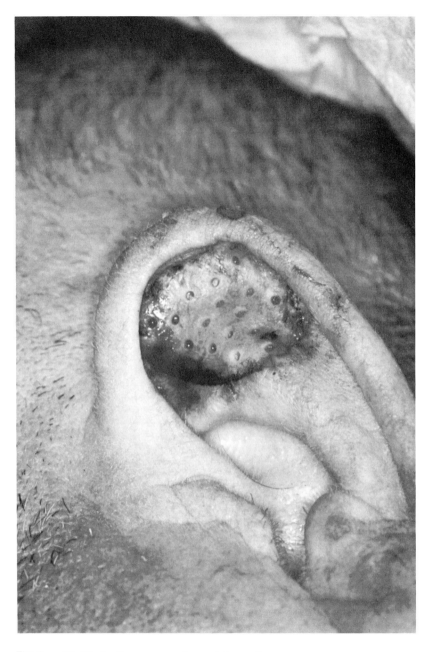

Fig 2. Multiple 2-mm punch excisions through the cartilage are made to speed up granulation time. (Courtesy of Dr. Roy Geronemus.)

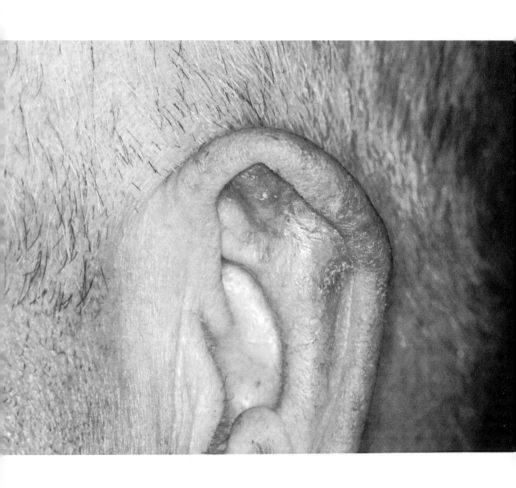

Fig 3.   The lesion was left to heal by second intention. Result is
         6 weeks postprocedure. (Courtesy of Dr. Roy Geronemus.)

PART V

SURGICAL PROCEDURES OF THE SCALP

DETERMINING BOUNDARIES OF THE "SAFE" DONOR AREA IN HAIR TRANSPLANTATION

By Samuel Ayres III, M.D.

Successful punch autografting for male pattern baldness depends on the principle of donor dominance. It is essential, therefore, that grafts not be harvested from donor sites on the occipital-parietal fringe that are 1) so high as to be subject to possible later hair loss in a patient whose eventual pattern is not yet apparent, or 2) so low as to be from areas of inherently poor density, again subject to eventual hair loss.

Good candidates have fringes of good hair density over a considerable width that become relatively sparse only in the lowest portion of the fringe. Poor candidates have fringes that are sparse throughout. Still other patients have moderate to good density only in the upper half or two-thirds of the fringe, often with drastically poorer density in the lower portion. In this last category, selecting areas of adequate density as donor sources is critical.

In addition, there are many technical causes of hair follicle destruction that may lead to poor growth of the graft. These include dull or eccentrically rotating punches, grafts not cut parallel to the hair shafts or not cut deeply enough, and overly zealous or careless trimming of the subcutaneous fat from the grafts. Excessively flaccid donor site skin will make harvesting of high-quality grafts much more difficult. To ensure good-quality grafts with a high yield of hairs per graft, harvesting must be done in areas of relatively high density, avoiding the low fringe area, where the density may be very sparse. In an effort to avoid taking grafts from areas too high on the fringe and presumably destined to future hair loss, the hair transplant surgeon may make the opposite and equally serious error of taking grafts from too low a site, where the hair is already sparse and will probably become even more so. A technique is described for determining the "safe" areas for donor sites.

TECHNIQUE

In patients with relatively early male pattern baldness, in whom the future pattern of loss is not yet evident, one can draw upon the experience of having seen many men with extensive male pattern baldness. The lowest (most posterior) extension of crown baldness, that is, the uppermost border of the permanent fringe, in the midline posteriorly, is approximately a finger's breadth above an imaginary line drawn across the posterior aspect of the scalp at the level of the tops of the ears, as viewed from behind (Fig 1). With this as a frame of reference, the typical arciform curve forming the superior border of the fringe along the posterolateral and lateral scalp must be imagined as an approximate guide in a relatively young patient. There are a number of extensively bald men in whom the posterior fringe extends higher in the midline posteriorly, resulting in a very wide fringe laterally as well as posteriorly. The reverse case, in which the fringe is substantially lower in the midline posteriorly, is almost by definition a case of very extensive early-onset male pattern baldness and a correspondingly low, narrow fringe, which is probably already quite evident at the time of initial presentation.

Therefore, the "finger's breadth above the tops of the ears" measurement has proven to be a useful starting point in most patients for identifying the upper margins of the "safe" fringe area. An additional aid in patients with early subtle thinning of the crown hair is wetting the hair. This helps to distinguish the area subject to continuing future hair loss from the permanent fringe hair by greatly accentuating the thinning, which may be scarcely apparent when the hair is dry (Fig 2). When the hair is wet, the division between thinning posterior crown hair and adjacent "safe" fringe hair frequently will be seen to confirm the "finger's breadth" rule.

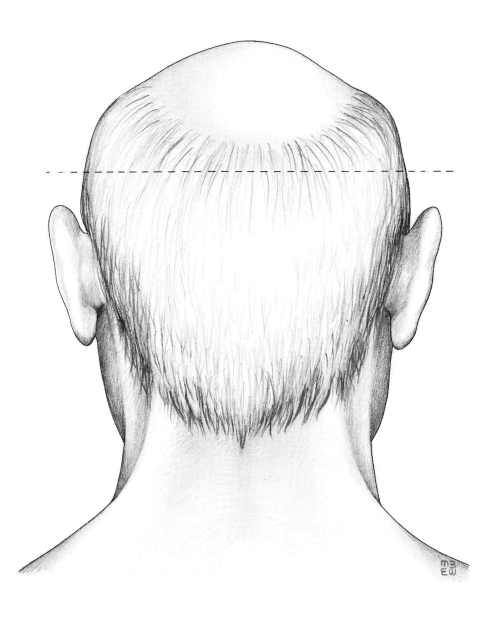

Fig 1. **The "finger's breadth above a line drawn (dashes) across the posterior aspect at the level of the tops of the ears."**

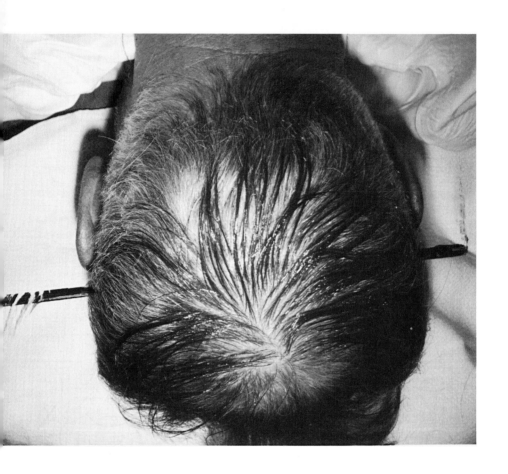

<u>Fig 2.</u> **Wetting the hair accentuates the thinning and helps to demarcate the permanent fringe.**

EXCISION OF SMALL SKIN LESIONS ON THE SCALP

By Marwali Harahap, M.D.

Excision of lesions on the scalp can result in profuse bleeding. This can be controlled by pressing the bleeding area against the underlying skull.

TECHNIQUE

The incision is marked out with gentian violet solution. Then the finger ring of a needle holder or other instrument can be placed firmly over the skin lesion, and the incision is made through it (Fig 1).

The ring is used to stretch the skin, allowing a neat vertical incision to be made and pressing the scalp against the underlying skull, which helps with hemostasis. Any additional bleeding prior to suturing can be controlled with electrocautery.

Often two layers of sutures are used in the scalp, one in the galea plane and one in the skin. However, one deep vertical mattress suture is usually sufficient (Fig 2).[1,2]

REFERENCES
1. Kyle J. Pye's Surgical Handicraft, 20th Ed. Bristol, UK, Wright Publishing Co, 1977, p 326.
2. Robinson JK. Wound closure by suturing. In Harahap M (ed): Principles of Dermatologic Plastic Surgery. New York, PMA Publishing Corp, 1988, p 41.

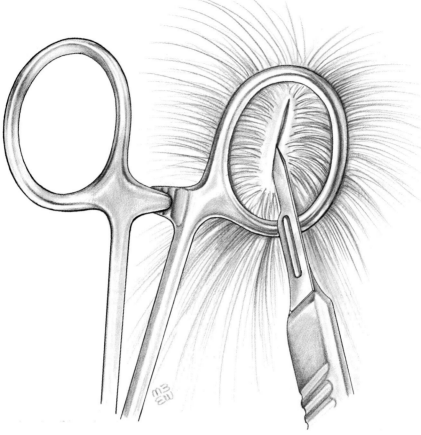

Fig 1. **The finger ring of a needle holder placed firmly over the skin lesion.**

Fig 2. **Suture in scalp lesion.**

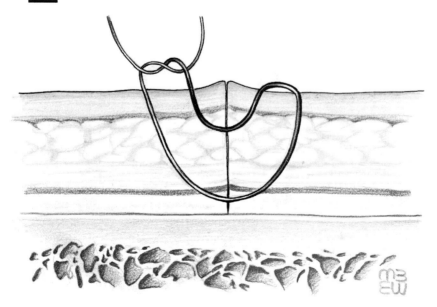

HAIR TRANSPLANTATION: VARIATIONS ON MINIREDUCTIONS

By Walter P. Unger, M.D.

In 1983, I described the use of minireductions as a simple adjunct to the regular-sized alopecia reductions.[1] They are also extraordinarily useful for repair sessions in people who have had poor transplanting, carried out—it is hoped—elsewhere, whom you are trying to repair but who are running out of grafts. Often a line of holes can be punched out at the same sites where grafts would have been used if they had been available, and instead of inserting grafts, the holes are simply closed with interrupted sutures (Figs 1 to 4). Such minireductions can either be done concomitantly with punch transplanting or may be done as small sessions on their own. They have the advantage of being able to follow any configuration, and the punch may be varied in size from 3 to 5 mm on the same line; that is, they may be tailor-made to fit hairless spaces.

Minireductions can also be used to save grafts by transplanting solid rows of hairs separated by untransplanted rows. The transplanted rows are done in two sessions, 4 months or more apart (Figs 5 to 8). The untransplanted rows are then punched out, and the gap is sutured closed (Figs 9 and 10) using a "Pierce-plasty."[2] In the vertex area of some patients I have been able on occasion to excise up to eighty 4.0- to 4.5-mm holes in a matter of 30 min. A small scar remains at the site of the excised line, and it is therefore not a suitable technique for dealing with every untransplanted line. However, substantial savings are possible in an individual who might refuse to consider regular alopecia reductions.

REFERENCES
1. Unger WP. Concomitant minireductions in punch hair transplanting. J Dermatol Surg Oncol 9:388–392, 1983.
2. Pierce HE. An improved method of closure of donor sites in hair transplantation. J Dermatol Surg Oncol 5:475–476, 1979.

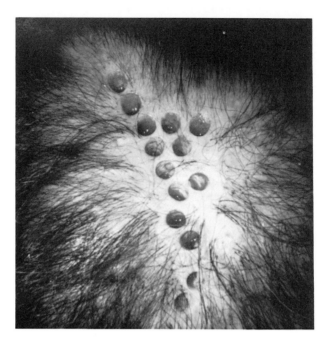

Fig 1. Fourteen sites have been punched out and removed using various sized punches corresponding to the size of the hairless spots.

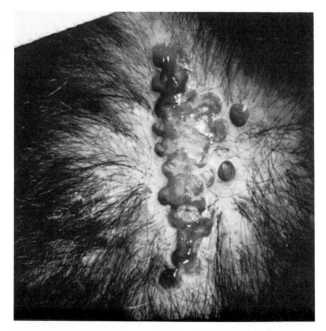

Fig 2. The "bridges" between holes have been cut, the intervening skin excised, and the area undermined for closure.

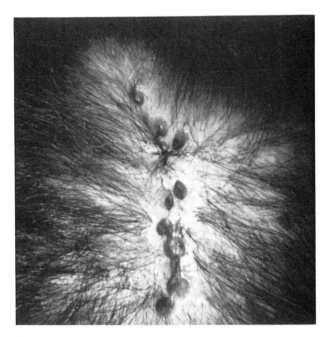

Fig 3.   **One suture in place.**

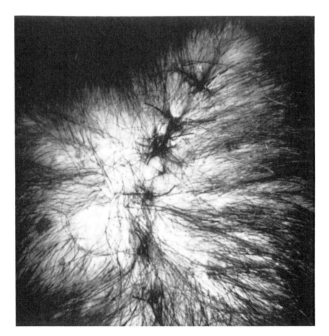

Fig 4.   **Closure completed with a total of six sutures. These sutures will be removed in 7 days.**

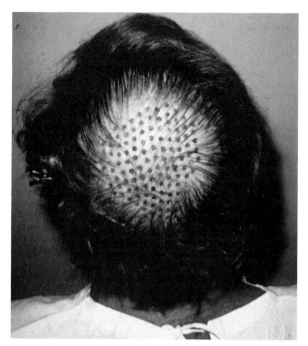

Fig 5.   **Pattern used for first and second session in vertex. Grafts were placed on same rows with sessions 4 months apart.**

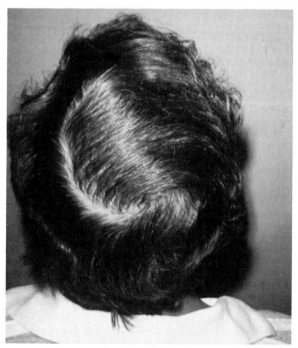

Fig 6.   **Growth of two sessions (240 plugs).**

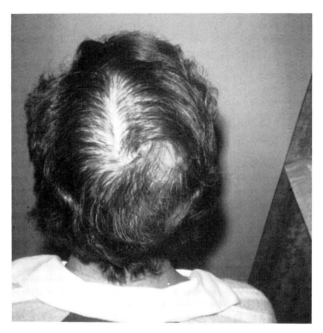

Fig 7. Hair parted at midline of previously transplanted vertex exposing a typical nontransplanted line of thinning hair between lines of transplanted hair.

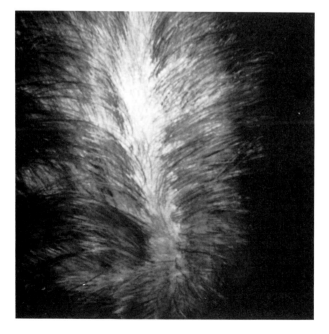

Fig 8. Close-up of Figure 7.

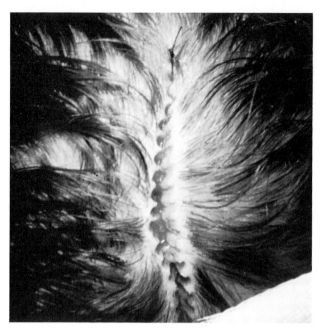

Fig 9.   A line of eighteen 4.5-mm sites has been punched out and removed from the thinning area. "Bridges" between the holes have been cut and one suture is in place to demonstrate the intended "z" closure ("Pierce-plasty").

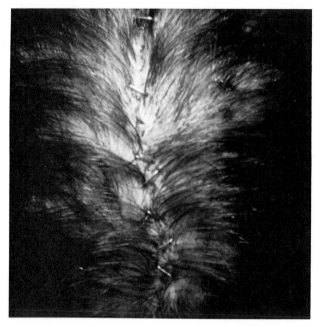

Fig 10.   Closure completed with the use of stainless steel staples.

REGIONAL ANESTHESIA FOR HAIR TRANSPLANTATION

By Thomas Kohn, M.D.

In performing anesthesia for hair transplantation, it is preferable to start with regional blockade of the supraorbital and supratrochlear nerves bilaterally. This will achieve complete anesthesia of the corresponding sides of the forehead and frontal area of the scalp to the lambdoidal suture and laterally to a line extending from the lateral portion of the eyebrow.

TECHNIQUE

A 3- to 5-ml amount of anesthetic solution, preferably 1% Xylocaine with epinephrine (Astra), is injected from the midline above the bridge of the nose laterally in a straight line just above the supraorbital rim for 3 cm. This is repeated on the other side for a bilateral block (Fig 1). Once anesthesia has been achieved, it is important to infiltrate 1% Xylocaine with epinephrine into the surgical site and laterally, extending to the extent of the proposed hairline, to achieve hemostasis.

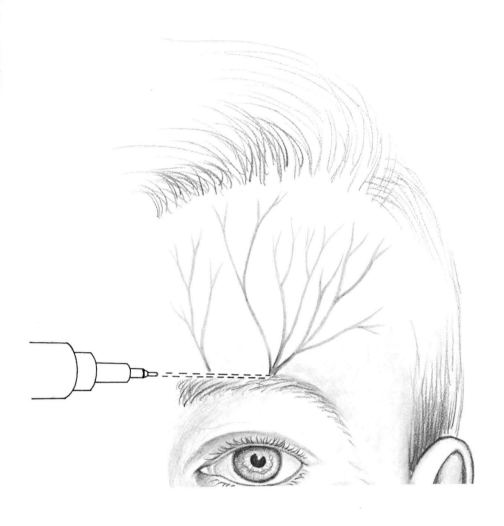

Fig 1.   Injection of anesthetic to achieve regional anesthesia of
         supraorbital and supratrochlear nerves.

SCALP REDUCTION TIPS

By James B. Pinski, M.D.

Two techniques employed during preparation of the scalp for surgery can simplify scalp reduction.

TECHNIQUES

A) Injection of saline prior to performing scalp reduction will delineate the galea from the periosteum, as the saline separates the two layers and simplifies undermining (Fig 1).

B) Bleeding of the wound edges in scalp reduction can be obviated by waiting a full 20 min following injection of Xylocaine with epinephrine (Astra). This allows maximal time for vasoconstriction to occur prior to surgery. With this technique, it is not necessary to use a Shaw scalpel.

C) Having cut one edge of the proposed reduction and undermined between the galea and periosteum in all directions, make a perpendicular excision at the widest point of the flap to be excised. Attach towel clips to the cut edges (Fig 2) and pull while pushing the remaining scalp in the opposite direction (Fig 3). This maneuver enables the surgeon to predetermine how much scalp can be excised prior to making the final cut. The problem of removing too much tissue and not being able to close the wound is avoided.

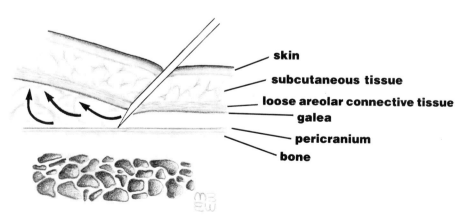

skin
subcutaneous tissue
loose areolar connective tissue
galea
pericranium
bone

Fig 1. Separation of the galea from the periosteum with saline.

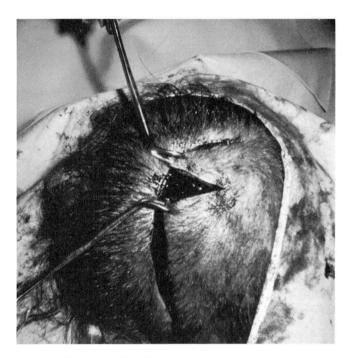

Fig 2.   Towel clips are attached to the cut edges.

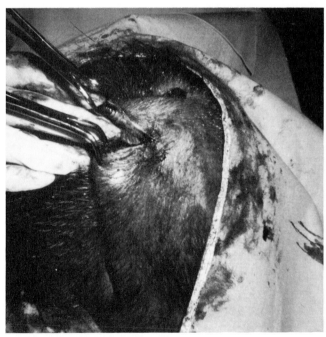

Fig 3.   The surgeon pulls one side while pushing the other side in
          the opposite direction.

PART VI

NAIL SURGERY

Nail Surgery
By Robert L. Baran, M.D.

Reconstruction of the Lateral Nail Fold After Lateral Longitudinal Nail Biopsy
By Eckart Haneke, M.D.

Segmental Matrix Excision for the Treatment of Ingrown Toenails
By Eckart Haneke, M.D.

NAIL SURGERY

By Robert L. Baran, M.D.

A number of techniques for nail surgery follow.

A) NAIL PLATE AVULSION

The classic technique for avulsion of the nail plate starts distally and proceeds proximally. An alternative technique is that of Cordero,[1] which starts proximally and proceeds distally. The latter is most useful when the pathology of the nail plate involves distal subungual hyperkeratosis and will be described here.

TECHNIQUE

A nail elevator is inserted below the proximal edge of the nail plate, which should be properly freed up at the corners (Fig 1). The root of the nail is placed on the proximal nail fold. The nail elevator can then be easily passed along the plane of cleavage between the lifted root of the nail (that does not adhere to the subungual matrix area) and the nail bed. The nail plate can then be pulled distally (Fig 2).

B) CHRONIC PARONYCHIA

Recalcitrant chronic paronychia may be an occupational disease caused by foreign bodies. It is found in hairdressers, people employed as dishwashers, and those engaged in milking of cattle. It often responds best to surgical intervention.[2]

TECHNIQUE

Surgical excision of a crescent-shaped piece of full-thickness skin, 5 mm at its greatest width and extending from one lateral fold to the other, is performed. It should include the entire swollen portion of the proximal nail fold. Some caution should be exercised with respect to depth of excision because of the insertion of the extensor tendon of the finger, which inserts into the terminal phalanx of this region (Fig 3). Healing is complete within 2 months.

C) NAIL MATRIX BIOPSY

Punch biopsy of the nail matrix does not require suturing if the diameter of the punch is no greater than 3 mm.

D) ACUTE SUBUNGUAL HEMATOMA AND NAIL BED LACERATION

Acute subungual hematoma involving more than 25% of the visible nail and/or nail bed laceration requires exploration of the nail bed and accurate approximation of the edges of the wound of the nail bed. The nail plate should be avulsed. The hematoma is evacuated, and any lacerations are sutured with absorbable suture material. After removal, the nail plate should have multiple holes drilled or burned through it. Then the nail plate should be replaced and held in place by nonabsorbable sutures passed through the fingertip and the distal free border of the nail. In an alternative method, the sutures pass through the lateral nail folds and the lateral edges of the nail (Fig 4).

The nail plate protects the repaired nail bed and serves as an exact and ideal template for it.

E) GUILLOTINE-TYPE INJURY

A guillotine-type injury of the nail bed, distal to the bony phalanx, may be allowed to heal by second intention with the expectation of a good functional and cosmetic result. This is especially true in infants (Fig 5).

REFERENCES
1. Cordero CFA. Ablacion ungueal: Su uso en la onycomycosis. Derm Int 14:21, 1965.
2. Baran R, Bureau H. Surgical treatment of recalcitrant chronic paronychias of the fingers. J Derm Surg Oncol 7:106–107, 1981.

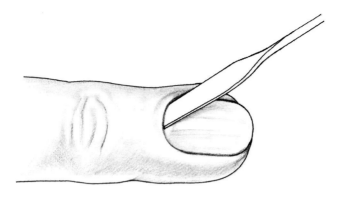

<u>Fig 1.</u> **Nail elevator in position.**

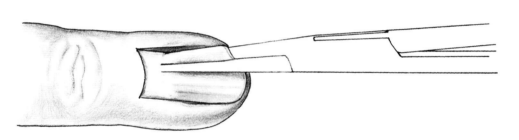

<u>Fig 2.</u> **Nail plate being pulled distally with forceps.**

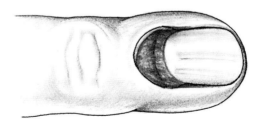

<u>Fig 3.</u> **Crescent-shaped excision of full-thickness skin in surgical treatment of chronic paronychia.**

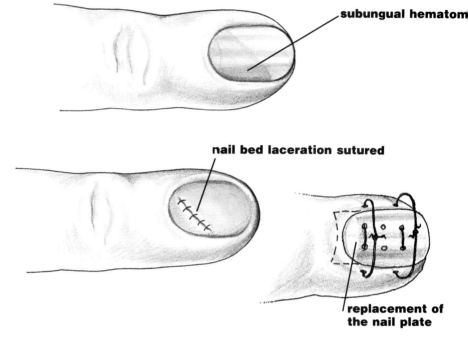

subungual hematoma

nail bed laceration sutured

replacement of the nail plate

Fig 4. Subungual hematoma (upper left). Nail bed laceration sutured following avulsion of nail plate (lower left), and replacement of nail plate, which has been drilled or burned with multiple holes.

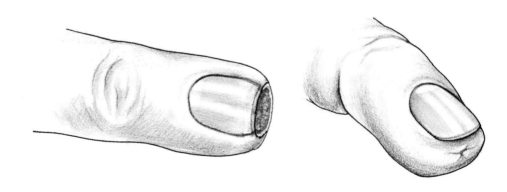

Fig 5. Guillotine-type injury (left); after healing (right).

RECONSTRUCTION OF THE LATERAL NAIL FOLD AFTER LATERAL LONGITUDINAL NAIL BIOPSY

By Eckart Haneke, M.D.

Many physicians are reluctant to perform nail biopsy, since they are afraid of cosmetically unacceptable scarring. The lateral longitudinal nail biopsy was introduced to minimize unwanted sequelae. This procedure results in a narrowing of the nail plate of only 2 to 3 mm. Suturing following longitudinal nail biopsy is often done by simple stitches running from the nail fold through the nail bed at the plate, but this produces an unacceptable loss of the lateral nail fold convexity (Fig 1).

To avoid this inversion of the lateral nail fold, a vertical mattress suture can be performed. The needle is inserted into the lateral aspect of the fingertip as far ventrally as possible; it is passed into the wound and then introduced into nail bed tissue and forced through the nail plate. The lateral nail fold is then again grasped with a fine forceps or skin hook in order to lift it, and the needle is passed through the dorsal aspect of the lateral nail fold. Tying the knot on the side of the lateral nail fold allows coaptation and elevation of the lateral nail fold and the nail plate, producing a natural and pleasing cosmetic result (Fig 2). Two or three of these sutures are usually sufficient. It should be noted that no sutures are passed through the nail matrix. It is advisable to remove sutures after 10 to 14 days.

Surgery of the nail and adjacent nail tissue requires full aseptic conditions because of the proximity to the distal phalanx. The use of a surgical glove with its fingertip cut away gives a sterile surrounding of the operative field.

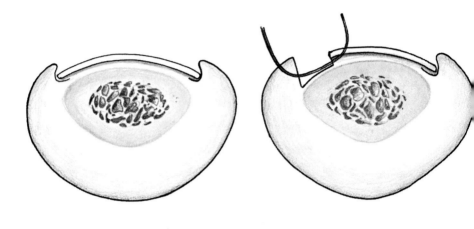

Fig 1. **Suturing with simple stitches after nail biopsy.**

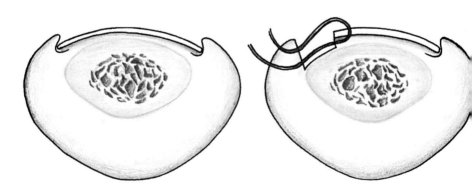

Fig 2. **Vertical mattress suture with the knot on the side of the lateral nail fold.**

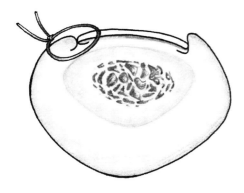

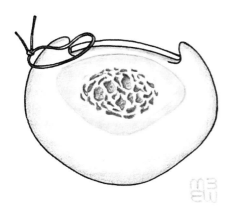

SEGMENTAL MATRIX EXCISION FOR THE TREATMENT OF INGROWN TOENAILS

By Eckart Haneke, M.D.

Ingrown toenails are very common. Many surgical treatment modalities have a very high recurrence rate. This is because the lateral matrix horn is not completely removed by most surgical procedures. Wedge excisions, for instance, invite recurrences because the very structure that is to be removed is the least well-exposed.

TECHNIQUE

A digital block is performed bilaterally. A 3- to 4-mm strip of ingrown toenail is excised using scissors. A 23-gauge needle is run along the lateral edge of the nail plate down to the base of the distal phalanx on the same side as the nail excision (Fig 1). Then a longitudinal or L-shaped incision is made on the lateral aspect of the proximal nail fold to expose the lateral matrix area, which is then dissected around the needle. The entire matrix horn is removed when tissue is seen to be all around the needle.

Hemostasis is achieved with topical hemostatic agents such as 30% aluminum chloride or light cautery. The wound is dressed with Vaseline (Chesebrough-Pond's) gauze and can be allowed to heal naturally.

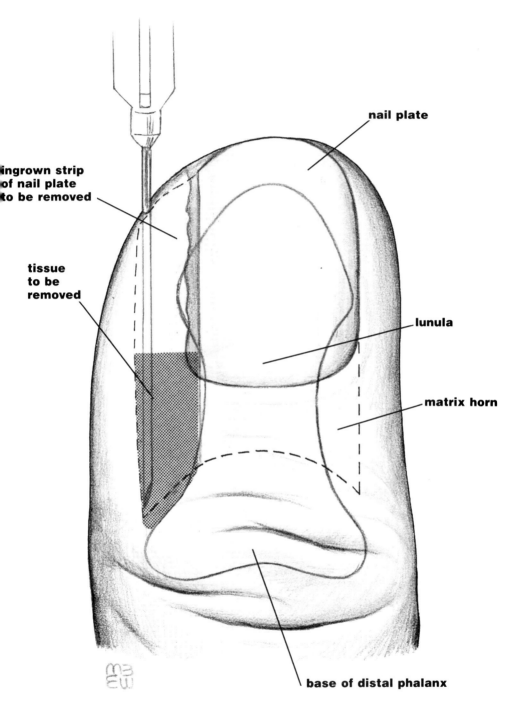

Fig 1. Needle run along base of distal phalanx on the same side
as excision.

PART VII

SURGICAL AIDS AND INSTRUMENTS

COTTON-TIPPED APPLICATORS USED IN CONJUNCTION WITH ELECTROCAUTERY FOR HEMOSTASIS

By Leonard Goldberg, M.D.,
Dan Meirson, M.D.,
and Perry Robins, M.D.

There are many methods to achieve hemostasis during cutaneous surgery. The more common ones include pressure applications of solutions, such as ferric subsulfate (Monsel's solution), 35% aluminum chloride, and trichloroacetic acid.[1] Other methods include spot coagulation using forceps and an electrocautery current or by the direct application of the electrocautery current to the bleeding vessel.[1] Another method of obtaining hemostasis by electrocoagulation after uncomplicated cutaneous surgery is described here.

TECHNIQUE

In this procedure, the bleeding surgical defect is completely filled with tightly packed cotton-tipped applicators (Fig 1). These are placed under pressure, with the cotton tips contiguous with each other. This direct pressure provides the dry field that is necessary for proper electrocautery when the applicators are removed.[2] The cotton applicators are then serially removed one at a time, and the vacated site is electrocoagulated (Figs 2 and 3). This simple method allows for rapid, complete, and permanent hemostasis in surgical wounds pending closure or healing by second intention.

REFERENCES
1. Goldberg L, Robins P. Hemostasis in cutaneous surgery. J Dermatol Surg Oncol 7:464–465, 1981.
2. Bennett RG. Fundamentals of Cutaneous Surgery. St. Louis, CV Mosby, 1988.

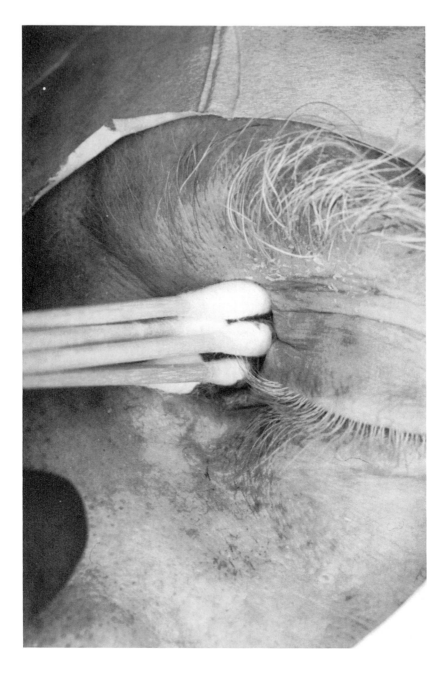

Fig 1. **Surgical defect filled with cotton-tipped applicators.**

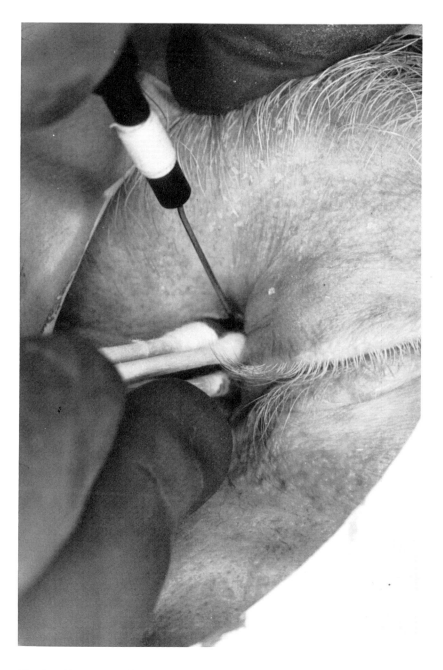

Fig 2. **Removal of applicators and electrocautery of the bleeding vessels.**

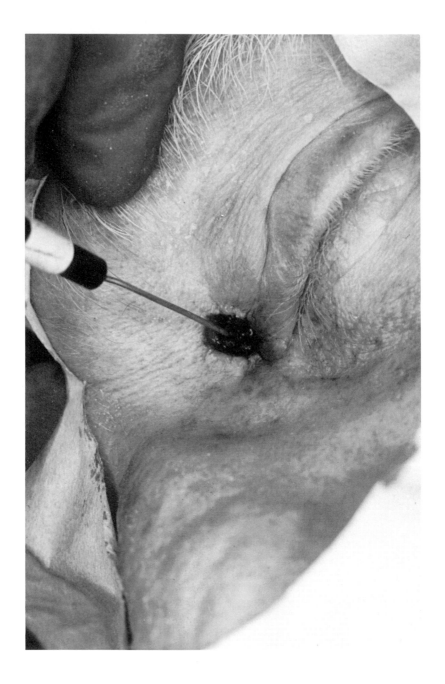

Fig 3.   **Surgical defect after hemostasis.**

FINDING, DEVELOPING, AND MAINTAINING A PROPER UNDERMINING PLANE

By Lawrence M. Field, M.D.

At what level is it appropriate to undermine? This question arises every time flap surgery of any type is performed. The surgeon might have absolute requirements for undermining at some precise depth, although a particular procedure might require specific graded and "stepped" levels of undermining.

Although Converse stated, "Incisions outlining the flap should be extended to the deep fascia whenever possible, and the flap should be raised by separating the fat from the fascia by sharp dissection,"[1] experience has shown that such a level of dissection is rarely necessary. Generally, the poorer the random circulation to the area, the thicker the flap must be. In well-vascularized areas, evolution of a flap containing dermal and subdermal plexi may well be sufficient. In facial surgery, McGregor believes "the appropriate level is just deep to the dermis, for any undercutting must be superficial to the level of the branches of the facial nerve."[2]

Rather than randomly selecting the level at which to begin undermining, the blunt ends of a needle holder[3] or, in special circumstances, the Iconoclast[4] (Luikart Surgical Supply) is appropriate for finding the most natural and relatively avascular separation plane. The use of a needle holder to start the process of undermining facilitates the undermining maneuver, because it finds the "proper line of cleavage for the dissection"[3] and leaves an appropriate and protective pad of subcutaneous fat on the flap undersurface, helping to prevent possible necrosis. Although the plane of cleavage between superficial and deep fascia seems appropriate,[2] this plane cannot always be anatomically localized. The bluntness of the needle holder dissection can be relied on to provide safety. In cervical-facial rhytidectomy, this surgeon has increasingly used both straight and curved suction cannulae with bluntly rounded tips for undermining after finding the proper entrance plane with the tips of the needle holder. These cannulae are especially useful in the dissecting process in the submental area, above the mandibular jowls, and, to some extent, the preauricular area.[5–7]

Where the skin is quite thin, as on the temple, in the periorbital and preauricular regions, the lower glabellar, proximal nose, the infravermilion chin, the supraclavicular torso, the neck, and the distal extremities, a small needle holder such as the Storz N5713 (Storz Instrument Co.) can be used. In locations where the evolving flaps are quite thick, as on the fatty frontal cheeks, back, abdomen, proximal extremities, and scalp, the Iconoclast can be used to spread the tissues after the proper plane has been found with the needle holder. The Iconoclast is especially useful in undermining between galea aponeurotica and the pericranium, sparing scalp follicles and preventing subsequent hair loss.[7] The initial use of the needle holder to locate the plane is shown schematically in Figure 1, the instruments themselves in Figures 2 and 3, the actual procedure exemplified by a forehead rotation flap in Figures 4 to 6, and the final closure in Figure 7.

Surgeons frequently dissect the undersurface of flaps with randomly directed movements. Even with the use of a curved undercutting scissors, the point of the scissor is often directed toward the surface rather than the curvature of the scissor oriented parallel to the curvature of the surface. The same point can be made for both convex and concave surfaces; that is, the curve of the undercutting instrument should conform with the surface anatomy (Fig 8). Further consideration must be made of the curvature of the surface on which a flap is being evolved, so the thickness of the flap remains constant or increases toward the base. As the depth of the dissection proceeds farther from the incised entrance point, the base of the flap should become thicker rather than thinner.

These simple rules will allow more precise approximation of the flap edges, lessen the potential for flap necrosis distal to an inadvertently thinned flap pedicle, and allow more precise recontouring.

Use of these instruments with excessive force may shear and inadvertently separate tissue attachments that should remain intact. The blunt, flat liposuction cannula is an ideal instrument with which to accomplish a remarkable degree of undermining and flap mobilization while leaving neurovascular septae between the subadjacent bed and the supradjacent flap intact.[8] As with all surgery, due caution and conservatism are appropriate.

REFERENCES
1. Converse JM. Plastic surgery and transplantation of skin. In Epstein E, Epstein E Jr (eds): Skin Surgery, 5th Ed, Vol I. Springfield, Ill, Charles C Thomas, 1982, p 266.
2. McGregor IA. Wound care. In Fundamental Techniques of Plastic Surgery and Their Surgical Applications, 3rd Ed. Baltimore, Williams & Wilkins, 1965, p 18.
3. Castanares S. Modifications of the face lift procedure. In Masters FW, Lewis JR Jr (eds): Symposium on Aesthetic Surgery of the Face, Eyelid, and Breast, Vol 4. Educational Foundation of the American Society of Plastic and Reconstructive Surgery. St. Louis, CV Mosby, 1972, pp 48–49.
4. Luikart R. The Iconoclast, a superb instrument for undermining. J Dermatol Surg Oncol 6:274–277, 1980.
5. Chrisman BC, Field LM. Facelift surgery up-date. J Dermatol Surg Oncol 10:544–548, 1984.
6. Field LM, Asken S, Caver C, et al. Liposuction surgery—a review. J Dermatol Surg Oncol 10:530–538, 1984.
7. Webster R, Pedroza F, Pedroza L, et al. The Iconoclast as an aid in blunt dissection of flaps of the scalp and forehead. J Dermatol Surg Oncol 8:793–795, 1982.
8. Field L, et al. Blunt liposuction cannula dissection with and without suction assisted lipectomy in reconstructive surgery. Submitted for publication.

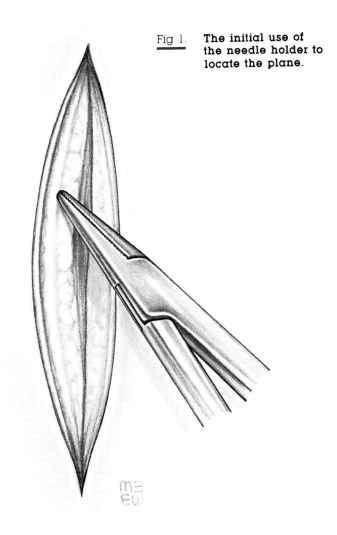

Fig 1. **The initial use of the needle holder to locate the plane.**

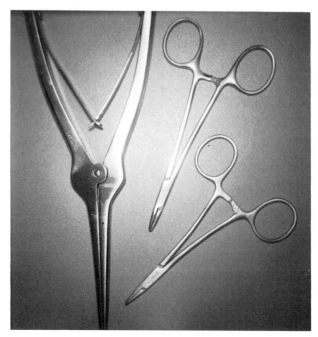

Fig 2.   The Luikart Iconoclast, the larger blunt-nosed Storz needle
holder N5700, and the narrower Storz needle holder N5713
(l–r).

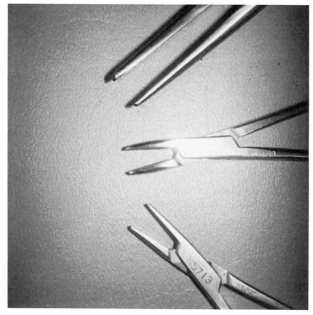

Fig 3.   The Iconoclast, the Storz N5700, and the Storz N5713, slightly
open.

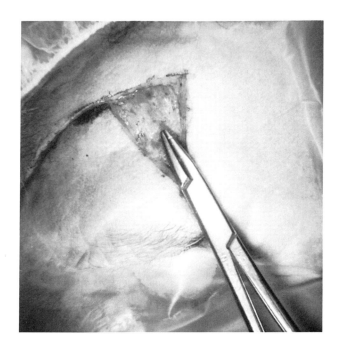

Fig 4. The blunt tip of the larger Storz needle holder positioned at the base of the flap to be developed.

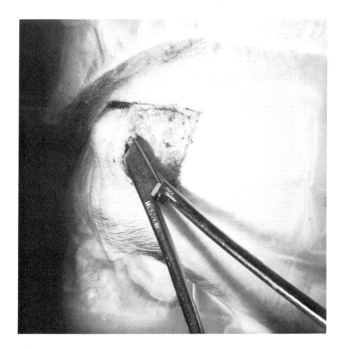

Fig 5. The base of the flap has been penetrated, with the instrument slightly open.

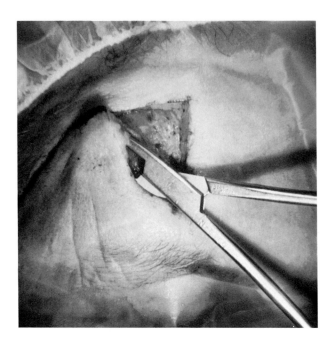

Fig 6.   **Blunt undermining is continued.**

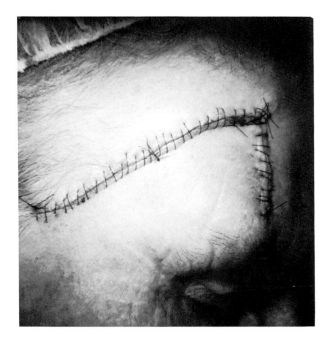

Fig 7.   **Closure of the advancement-rotation flap.**

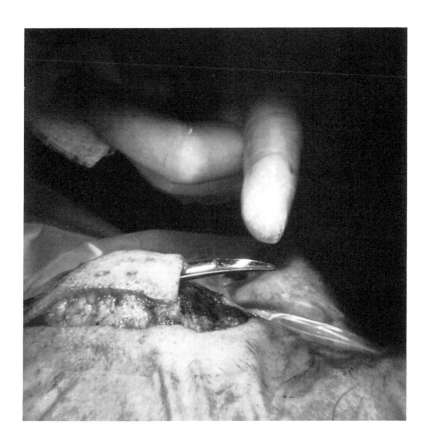

Fig 8.   **Curved undermining scissors within a subcutaneous tunnel, which is parallel with the convex flap surface.**

OUTER TABLE SLING SUTURE

By Janis P. Campbell, M.D.,
Richard G. Glogau, M.D.,
Samuel J. Stegman, M.D.,
and Theodore A. Tromovitch, M.D.

Cutaneous carcinomas located on the temple and forehead regions often prove to be extensive lesions when excised by microscopically controlled surgery.[1] Resection of these carcinomas frequently results in removal of the frontalis muscle and fascia down to the periosteum. Loss of muscle and nerve leaves the patient unable to raise the eyebrow, and it often droops over the upper lid. Closure of the wound by skin grafting or healing by second intention does not correct the eyebrow droop. We describe here a technique, the outer table sling suture, to correct this eyebrow droop.

TECHNIQUE

Using a sterilized hand drill, make two openings through the outer table of the frontal bone above the eyebrow. The openings are spaced at a proper distance to accommodate the arc of the suture needle entering and exiting the holes. Passage of the needle is facilitated if the holes are drilled at a 45° angle from the outer table toward the adjacent opening (Fig 1, insert). A nonabsorbable suture such as Mersilene (Ethicon) or Supramid (S. Jackson Inc.) is used. The needle tip is passed in and out of the two holes in the outer table and subsequently through the deep dermis of the eyebrow tissue. The suture is tied to align the eyebrow with the height of the eyebrow on the contralateral side (Fig 1). The holes are sealed with bone wax. The wound can be left to heal by second intention, or if split-thickness skin grafting is contemplated and a suitable recipient bed exists, the graft can be applied immediately. However, if the recipient site is unsatisfactory, for example, greater than 1 cm of bone is exposed, the wound can be left to granulate for a few weeks, and grafted later. When this suture technique is used at initial closure, it often eliminates the need for a secondary procedure to realign the eyebrow.

A manual drill is used rather than a motor-driven drill because the loss of resistance that occurs as the metal bit penetrates the outer table and enters the diploe is more pronounced. Another useful clue to penetration of the diploe is the appearance of a blood-red tinge in the bone shavings from the drill. The use of bone wax prevents desiccation of the diploe and inner table of bone, and prophylactic antibiotics provide protection against infection.

REFERENCE
1. Carruther JA, Stegman SJ, Tromovitch TA, et al. Basal cell carcinomas of the temple. J Dermatol Surg Oncol 9:759–762, 1983.

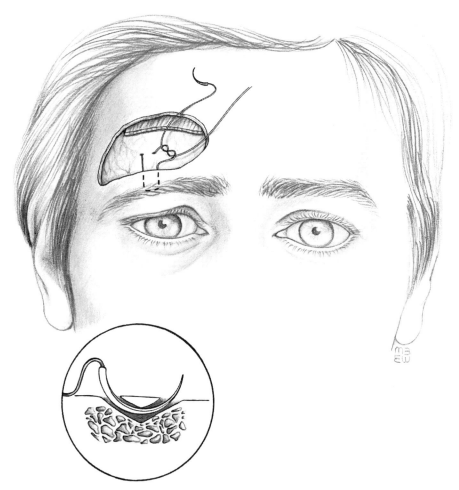

Fig 1.   Holes drilled into the outer table of the frontal bone spaced so that they accommodate the arc of the needle (see insert). Suture is passed through dermis of eyebrow.

RATIONAL USE OF ABSORBABLE SUTURE

By C. William Hanke, M.D.

A tenet of good excisional technique is the closure of subcutaneous dead space. Absorbable suture materials are used to close dead space to reduce the incidence of hematoma, infection, and wound dehiscence.

Polyglactin 910 (Vicryl, made by Ethicon) and polyglycolic acid (Dexon, Davis & Geck) are the two absorbable sutures used most commonly for this purpose. It is important to remember that absorbable sutures are foreign materials even though they are eventually degraded. The use of excessive amounts of absorbable suture material can contribute to less than optimum results.

TECHNIQUE

When using absorbable sutures, select the smallest caliber absorbable suture that will provide tensile strength sufficient for closing the wound. No more than three knots should be tied in order to minimize the amount of suture that is buried. No additional absorbable sutures other than those necessary to close the dead space should be used. These recommendations are based on an unpublished study undertaken by the author, which showed that use of large caliber suture materials with greater than three knots increases risks and prolongs the wound healing process (Figs 1 to 4).

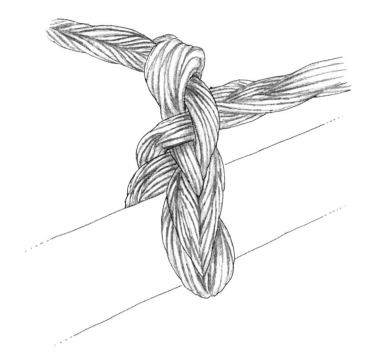

Fig 1.   **Rendering of 4-0 Polyglactin 910 tied to a stainless steel post using 3 knots (40×).**

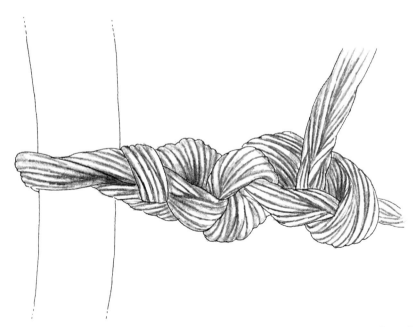

Fig 2.   **Rendering of 4-0 Polyglactin 910 tied to a stainless steel post using 5 knots (40×).**

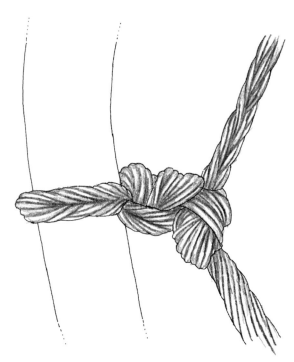

Fig 3. **Rendering of 5-0 Polyglactin 910 tied to a stainless steel post using 3 knots (40×).**

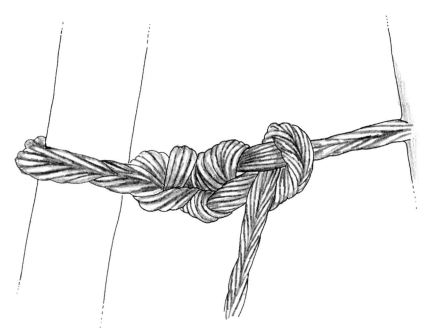

Fig 4. **Rendering of 5-0 Polyglactin 910 tied to a stainless steel post using 5 knots (40×).**

RETRACTION SUTURES IN EYELID SURGERY

By Ricardo G. Mora, M.D.

For working on lesions adjacent to the free margin of the lower eyelid with techniques such as Mohs micrographic surgery or full-thickness wedge excision, retraction sutures pull the eyelid away from the globe and allow excellent visualization with relative immobilization. This technique is superior to the use of a chalazion clamp, which often hinders access.

TECHNIQUE

Sutures are placed through the eyelid margin both lateral and medial to the lesion to be excised (Fig 1a). The sutures are pulled away from the globe and up by the nurse or assistant. This allows excellent exposure and provides safety for the globe (Fig 1b). At the completion of the surgical procedure, the sutures are removed.

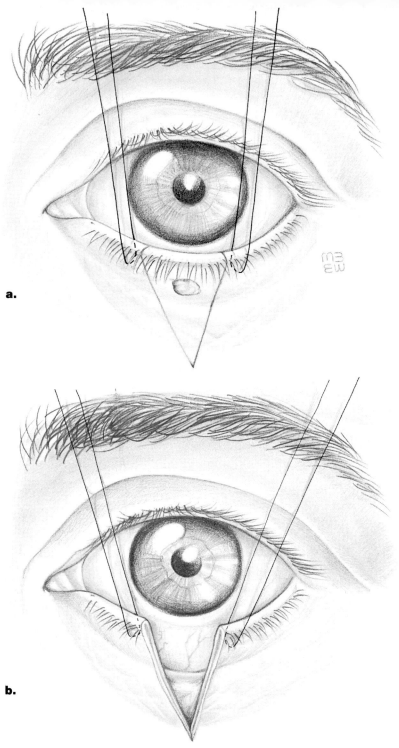

a.

b.

Fig 1.   Sutures placed through the eyelid margin used to expose the
         globe.

INDEX

Flaps:
  rhombic, 30–31
  undermining plane for, 103–9

Gibbs, Richard, 3
Glogau, Richard G., 110
Goldberg, Leonard, 99
Granulation tissue, curettage of, 38–41
Guillotine injury of nail bed, 88

Hair transplantation:
  anesthesia for, regional, 81–82
  minireductions and, 75–80
  "safe" donor area for, 69–72
Hand, dermabrasion of, 45–46
Haneke, Eckart, 91, 94
Hanke, C. William, 112
Harahap, Marwali, 73
Helical reconstruction, 60–62
Hematoma, subungual, 88, 90
Hemostasis, cotton-tipped
  applicators with
  electrocautery for, 99–102
Hernández-Pérez, Enrique, 28
Hyperhidrosis, 32–35

Ice-pick scars, punch float technique
  for, 47–49

Kohn, Thomas, 8, 81
Kuflik, Emanuel G., 53

Meirson, Dan, 99
Mikhail, George R., 22
Mobile skin, shave technique for, 24–25
Mora, Ricardo G., 115
Mouth, biopsy of, 15–17
M-plasty, 26–27

Nails:
  avulsion of, 87, 89
  biopsy of, 88
    reconstruction after, 91–93
  guillotine injury of, 88, 90
  hematoma and laceration of, 88
  inflammation of, 87, 89
  ingrown, segmental matrix
    excision for, 94–95
Nevi:
  punch biopsy for, 28–29
  shave technique for, 24–25
Nose, anesthetic injection into, 6

Oral biopsy, 15–17
Orentreich, David S., 54

Orentreich, Norman, 54
Outer table sling sutures, 110–11

Paronychia, 87, 89
Pinski, James B., 83
Pitard, Edward F., 47
Plantar skin, anesthetizing, 3–5
Punch biopsy, nevi removed by, 28–29
Punch excision, ear cartilage, 63–66
Punch float technique, 47–49
Punch graft, earlobe, facial scar
  revision with, 54–59

Ratz, John L., 50
Retraction sutures for eyelid, 115–16
Reyes, Blas A., 38
Rhombic flap, 30–31
Robins, Perry, 18, 38, 63, 99

Scalp:
  excision of lesions on, 73–74
  hair transplantation. See Hair
    transplantation.
  minireductions of, 75–80
  reduction tips, 83–84
Scars:
  ice-pick, punch float technique
    for, 47–49
  revision of facial, with punch
    graft from earlobe, 54–59
Scherrer-Koch, Annalis, 32
Sclerotic basal cell carcinoma,
    margin definition of, 22–23
Shave technique for nevi, 24–25
Sling suture, outer table, 110–11
Sole, anesthetizing, 3–5
Stegman, Samuel J., 110
Sutures:
  absorbable, 112–14
  outer table sling, 110–11
  retraction, for eyelid, 115–16

Thin skin, shave excision of, 24–25
Toenails, ingrown, segmental
  excision for, 94–95
Tromovitch, Theodore A., 110

Undermining plane, 103–9
Unger, Walter P., 75

Vigilon dressing, 50
Vinciullo, Carl, 30

Wheeland, Ronald G., 10

Yarborough, John M., Jr., 47